The Pilot's Manual of Medical Certification and Health Maintenance.

Richard O. Reinhart, M.D.
U.S.A.F. Flight Surgeon
Sr. FAA AME

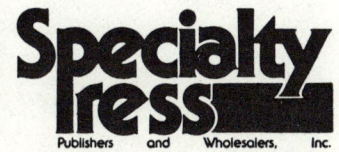

© 1982 Richard O. Reinhart, M.D.
All rights reserved. No part of this publication may be reproduced without prior written permission from the publisher.

Printed in the United States of America
10 9 8 7 6 5 4 3 2 1

ISBN 0-933424-36-1 (softbound edition)
ISBN 0-933424-38-8 (hardbound edition)

LC #82-62124 (softbound edition)
LC #82-062124 (hardbound edition)

Published by: Specialty Press Publishers & Whoesalers, Inc.
Box 426, 729 Prospect Avenue
Osceola, Wisconsin 54020

Dedication:

To my wife Marcia
and to my
Sons, Mark and Curtis

Acknowledgments:

My sincere thanks go to those around me who have been supportive in this new venture of writing. The encouragement of Larry Medin, the pilot's viewpoint of Pat Boab, and aeromedical assistance from Drs. Carter, Hodgson, and Gullett, and of course the work of Sharon Hanks in her chapter, were all instrumental in the final achievement of this book.

Contents

		Page
Preface		1
Introduction		4
One	The Philosophy of Pilot Health Monitoring and Health Maintenance	8
Two	Disqualifying Medical Conditions	16
Three	The FAA's Certification Process	29
Four	Specific Health Problems and Flying	56
Five	How to Work With Your Family Doctor and Your AME	76
Six	A Pilot's Own Health Maintenance Program	85
Seven	Airworthy Anatomy by Sharon M. Hanks	91
Eight	An Exercise Program for Pilots	116
Nine	Habits and Abuses that Affect Your Certification, and Miscellaneous Medical Topics	122
Appendix I	Part 67 of Federal Air Regulations	131
Appendix II	Conditions for which the Medical Certificate Will Be Denied or Deffered	140
Index		168

Preface

"PEOPLE WHO LIVE IN FEAR of disease are apt to become ill. Anxiety quickly demoralizes the whole body and lays it open to illness and disease. . ." This statement, made by James Allen in the 1800's in *As a Man Thinketh,* describes the feeling and predicament of many professional pilots. They are not satisfied with the way they feel or are concerned about their careers, but are justifiably apprehensive about what to do to feel better or maintain their health without jeopardizing their careers.

As a result, the medical certification process of pilots, especially those who earn a living by flying, is an emotional, personal, lonely, and often threatening experience. The process is misunderstood and feared by all except by those sitting in judgment, is viewed by the healthy as a nuisance, and is thought by many to create more problems than it resolves. Yet, if used effectively, this unavoidable process should be of benefit, not only to the individual pilot, but to the entire aviation industry and to those who use it.

With a pilot's own career and his employer's investment in him at stake, it is frustrating for me to realize that despite the incentive to keep flying, few pilots truly want to understand or respect the process of medical certification or health maintenance. It appears that only those pilots who have lost their medical certification become concerned about discussing the subject, and they are, of course, understandably angry, defensive and confused. The threat of being grounded, the misunderstanding of the certification process, plus the pilot's ignorance about his *true* health status can often add to the anxiety associated with an unexplained pain or change in how he feels. This added, yet unnecessary, fear often interrupts the job and joy of flying. Comrades, in an admirable desire to help, use misleading "war stories" to describe their own interpretation of certification, often compounding the pilot's dilemma.

To my knowledge, no book addresses the all-important certification process—certainly no book written for pilots by a pilot who is also a physician and an Aviation Medical Examiner (AME). Well-meaning articles appear in trade journals, Federal Aviation Administration (FAA) publications, and company and union news letters, but I have yet to see a comprehensive discussion and explanation of the entire certification process including the medical standards that *pilots* are expected to meet. **A pilot's greatest fear is a medical condition of any degree of significance being prematurely reported to the FAA, causing him to lose control of his career.** Yet little has been written on what the pilot realistically can do *on his own* to protect his health and his medical certificate. I hope this book will provide that knowledge and instruct you, the pilot, in the procedures and guidelines used by your AME and the FAA. Most importantly, the book will discuss the development of your own health-maintenance program.

This book is intended primarily for professional pilots, since they must meet the strictest medical standards and because they have the greatest responsibility in the air when they are medically certified (and the most to lose if they flunk the physical exam). The concept, however, is the same for any pilot who wants to maintain his or her health and medical certification. Fortunately for the professional pilot, he has an all-important motivating factor in his favor to stay healthy—his career! No other professional person is so dependent on proving good health to his boss and to a government agency.

The philosophy expressed here is my own and is not meant to interfere with or erode an acceptable health-maintenance program that an individual pilot may already be following. My personal comments and opinions are addressed to those pilots who are, or feel that they are, aeromedically neglected.

Neither is this book meant to be a dissertation on any scientific medical study. It purposely avoids many sides of the subject, but, at the same time, is an attempt to *define* the issue for the pilot. To my colleagues in aviation medical departments who want to keep their pilots healthy and flying, and to help those who have problems: I share your frustration in coping with the misunderstandings of your professional goals. The occasional opinion that flight surgeons or aviation doctors are "out to get" the pilot should have disappeared at the same time that it was realized that mechanics could fix airplanes just as well as pilots—or better. To the concerned pilot who has picked up this book: I hope I may give you some facts with which to challenge the rumors you hear and enable you to permit us to do our job of helping pilots. There is nothing new or unique, nothing "revolutionary" in my program for pilots. I only hope to clarify the multitude of misconceptions concerning medical certification and health maintenance. Misinformation puts you at the mercy of the AME and the FAA. However, by becoming familiar with the whole process of your medical cer-

Preface

tification, you won't need the FAA to force you to be healthy. Instead, you can keep a step ahead of the FAA by using the same medical tools that the AME and the FAA use and, as a result, actually assist your AME or private medical doctor in keeping you certified. Being in control is what you enjoy about flying. You can also take control of your medical status and medical certificate. You don't have to blindly depend on your doctor and the bureaucracy to keep you flying.

The simple objective of this book is to provide you, the pilot, with the medical and administrative tools to protect your health and your medical certificate for as long as possible. I am confident that with this added knowledge *you* can greatly improve your odds of not being forced into an early medical retirement.

Richard O. Reinhart, M.D.

Introduction

PROFESSIONAL PILOTS—corporate, airline, charter, military or instructor—have the potential to lose more by having an annual physical examination than any other professional, since pilots know there is a possibility the exam will *keep* them from flying. Yet the person who earns a living flying airplanes and people through the sky has a better opportunity to maintain a desired healthy status than any other worker because he or she came to the profession in near perfect health, and that health has been monitored frequently.

Why do a significant percentage of professional pilots never reach retirement? How can so many "healthy" pilots be medically grounded for months and even years before being returned to flying status? With a career at stake, why do professional pilots abuse their health and fail to follow the advice of doctors and other medical experts and consultants who are trying to keep them healthy and certified?

The answers to these questions are basically simple: apathy, laziness and ignorance—all leading to fear and mistrust. Apathy about the urgency of maintaining health; laziness or procrastination in pursuing a good health-maintenance program; and ignorance or lack of understanding of one's medical status and the FAA's medical certification process. Put another way, pilots have frequent contact with health care and its principles, but many do not take advantage of this valuable resource. They don't know how, or—worse yet—they are afraid.

Professional pilots, like the rest of us, always fear that something serious will be found unexpectedly during an exam, especially if they have symptoms, even minimal ones. Unlike most of us, however, a pilot fears that the doc will find something wrong when he is feeling great and has *no* symptoms. In addition, the pilot fears that even if his family doctor and his AME prove he *is* healthy, the paperwork will get screwed up somewhere in the bureaucracy—and it can. In each of these situations, not only is the pilot's health in question, but his *career* is threatened.

Introduction

Yet, despite potentially "losing" as a result of the annual (or semi-annual) exam, professional pilots also are fortunate in terms of their ability to *control* their health. Let me illustrate by stating some known and accepted conditions of a professional pilot's life style. As an instrument-rated commercial pilot, a flight surgeon for the Minnesota Air National Guard, and a practitioner of aviation medicine and aeromedical certification, I am in regular, direct contact with professional pilots and am speaking from several perspectives of relevant experience. Let's examine some special characteristics of pilots as a *subculture* within our working society.

Professional pilots are inherently healthy. Initially, to be hired, pilots are medically screened from many applicants, most of whom were already healthier than the majority of their non-aviator friends. Therefore, before even beginning this career, practically all chronic diseases were proven to be absent. This, along with feeling good, gives the pilot a secure sense of being in good health, even though the feeling may be unwarranted.

A professional pilot's health is monitored periodically to insure continued good health. Every six or twelve months the pilot must prove to the FAA (and himself) the absence of any major illness or potentially incapacitating medical problem. Granted, the FAA physical is no more beneficial than the doctor giving the exam. We both know that there are exams and then there are *exams;* and the results can be handled in a multitude of ways. Some results are mishandled and, therefore, are not acceptable to the pilot being examined nor in the best interests of aviation. Yet, the fact remains, as a pilot you have had a medical evaluation every six to twelve months and this puts you miles and years ahead of most Americans.

A professional pilot has the strongest motivation to maintain his health: the preservation of his career! Despite this stimulus—but armed with apathy and complacency (and some unrealistic feelings of invincibility)—the typical professional pilot does one of four things regarding his health and medical certification:

1. Pursues a good health-maintenance program, consequently greatly improving the probability of retaining a medical certificate.

2. Respects and trusts the FAA examiner and seeks his help after any medical problem arises, but does little to practice a health *maintenance* program for himself.

3. Does not respect or trust the FAA examiner, but gets certified by him "because he's done it for me for years without any questions." The pilot then seeks help from another doctor (usually not experienced in aviation medicine) for medical problems. Unfortunately, many of these doctors have little knowledge of the flying profession and how "usual and customary medical care" affects your FAA medical certification, flying responsibilities, and career.

4. Merely gets by the FAA exam (with fingers crossed) and waits out the next six months hoping nothing develops. This is especially common among older pilots who feel secure in their job. The philosophy is to worry about a medical grounding only if and when it happens. In other words, the idea is to avoid making waves—this guy will worry about his health when he retires.

A professional pilot has the time and the money to pursue a worthwhile health-maintenance program. The FAA exam is not usually adequate in monitoring and maintaining a pilot's health. To be beneficial, it needs to be a comprehensive medical evaluation with subsequent correction of problems and assistance in learning basic medical principles. However, most of the time and money in *anyone's* budget is not put to medical use until a tangible and immediate need arises. Often there seem to be higher-priority needs for the pilot's time and money—until he is grounded. *Then* there is no limit to the measures a pilot will pursue to unravel his dilemma. This predicament invariably occurs years *after* the medical problem could have been resolved or prevented. Most professional pilots really need to sit back and say, "Hey, I'm not as healthy, as I could be. My career isn't that secure, and my loss-of-license insurance isn't the answer if I develop a medical problem." Time and money spent on health maintenance now are the best ways to secure your future.

The professional pilot has vast resources with which to educate himself in health maintenance. Most professional pilots are well informed, but they are not physicians. Much of their medical information, therefore, is found in the lay press, which relates to the general population. The advice usually does not consider the unique and restrictive medical criteria to which a professional pilot must adhere; consequently this well-intended advice is of questionable usefulness. To add to the confusion, there are conflicting professional viewpoints within the health profession on very basic and fundamental health habits. Yet, pilots are continually reading and exchanging new thoughts among themselves about nutrition, physical conditioning and health maintenance. How much of this sometimes overwhelming information is beneficial and understood—and how to apply it—is another matter. For health education the prudent pilot can and should turn to his flight physician for information, just as he would turn to an aircraft mechanic for airplane maintenance.

Some professional pilots can depend on an organization or union for assistance when medical trouble develops or medical certification is lost. Such support by a peer organization often reinforces apathy and a false sense of security. Valuable as these groups may be in restoring certification, they are already behind the wall of red tape, an obstacle which must be overcome even before they can start to re-

Introduction

solve the pilot's individual difficulty. Much credit is due their efforts, but I'm sure that an all too common feeling is "if only I had done something to prevent or find this problem earlier." "If only" are two mighty small words when it comes to restoring your medical certification. Ultimately, with or without organizational support, the pilot is still fighting this battle alone.

The professional pilot has "clout" enabling him to change his working environment, improve his performance and preserve his medical flying status. Flying people in "friendly skies" is a major responsibility for pilot *and* management. It is unlikely that either side would irresponsibly ignore legitimate suggestions for improving the achievement of this basic goal of keeping aircraft and pilots flying safely. However, the intent of a change can be misinterpreted or get bogged down in petty bureaucratic and personal goals so that the objective is lost in the shuffle. The result in the aviation business, unfortunately, is sometimes a defensive attitude by management, the FAA, or the pilot group, whereby this "clout" is used negatively as a weapon, rather than being positive and constructive.

From the foregoing it is clear that the individual pilot does, in fact, have more control over his medical destiny than he might realize or be willing to accept — providing the pilot can cope with those who will be judging him.

So what to do? You are one against a system, with a career at stake, required to work with complex and frequently misunderstood aeromedical rules and regulations. Your medical status is not understood by some non-aviation doctors who are misinformed about FAA protocol and can lead you into the FAA's red tape. And you expect that if you are not healthy, you will be reported immediately to the FAA and grounded. Yet, you have the best odds of staying healthy and certified if you are willing to accept the responsibility of controlling your medical status.

I hope to show that there are many factors you alone can control for your benefit as an aviator, to better the odds of maintaining satisfactory health for yourself, your employer, and the FAA. There are no magic solutions — though the means are simple and basic. I will not attempt to imply that my health maintenance program will guarantee you a flying career until age 60. I will, however, guide you through a program that is realistic, factual and adaptable to your specific responsibilities.

You *do* have control over your medical future and flying career! Take control *now* — don't wait to reach for the stick *after* things start falling apart!

1

The Philosophy of Pilot Health Monitoring and Health Maintenance

Consider: You're at lunch before a turn-around trip . . .

"Hey George, what do you think? *My* family doc gave me some pills to take because he said my blood pressure is up a bit. I don't think he knows I'm a pilot. What should I do?"

George: "Don't sweat it, Fred. Just don't say anything at your FAA exam and hope your blood pressure is OK."

Or: over a beer at the end of a trip . . .

"Jack, I've been meaning to ask you . . . I took an insurance exam and they said there was something wrong with my urine. My FAA physical is due next month. What the hell should I do?"

Jack: "No problem, Fred. See *my* examiner. He never checks my urine and, in fact, really doesn't do much at all. That's why I see him. Why rock the boat—RIGHT?"

WHY *LOOK* FOR A PROBLEM when you're feeling fine? Besides, why not wait until something goes wrong and then tell the family doc? Why say anything to the FAA if *you* think you're OK? Isn't this they way the majority of pilots reason when discussing their medical certification?

But when it comes to your airplane, you have a different set of values and priorities. Do you not *actively* seek out a problem or potential malfunction even if you know the bird is flying well? You preflight, you follow checklists, you subject your flying machine to periodic exams. Next to maintaining your flying proficiency, you are most possessive about maintaining the airworthiness of the aircraft you fly.

There is a valid reason for the FAA health-monitoring program. However, fear and skepticism about the FAA and its medical exams come from misunderstanding of the medical certification process and the impact of some medical problems on flying safely. By comparing the generally accepted practice of periodic maintenance inspection of

Health Maintenance

your aircraft with the practice of *health* maintenance, I hope to clarify the philosophy of your required FAA medical exam.

It seems to me that your "human machine" deserves no less concern and maintenance than your flying machine. I am certain that *all* responsible pilots would welcome the resources with which to provide themselves the same level of maintenance of their health as they already willingly expect will be provided their aircraft. Why doesn't it happen? Because of the fear of losing one's career once one's health status is reported to the FAA.

No intelligent pilot would fly if he knew he had a problem that would suddenly incapacitate him or create a distraction on the flight deck. An approach to minimums in turbulence is not the time to have your buddy cry out in pain or faint! Contrary to popular belief, and *medically* speaking, your company, your doctors, and the FAA have only one goal: to keep you healthy and free of disability or distracting medical problems—to keep you flying safely. Is that any different than your philosophy on the responsibilities of flying? There shouldn't be two standards.

Now that we agree on this basic philosophy, let's all rush to our FAA examiner and say, "Hey Doc, see if I've got any problem which is going to make me unsafe to fly." Why the chuckles! Did I hear somebody say, "No Way!" Obviously, in spite of all of our well-intentioned objectives, the environment that would *encourage* pilots to seek their personal "preventive maintenance"—as in airplane maintenance—just doesn't exist.

Why not?

It's difficult, if not impossible, to explain to each pilot's satisfaction the purpose of health *monitoring* for a pilot who already feels okay: "How can I have a disqualifying problem if I don't feel sick?" He is challenged by well-established contradictions, misconceptions, historically poor medical evaluations and follow-ups, plus "testimonials" that would discredit most attempts to justify even the best intentions of FAA examiners, family doctors and flight surgeons. So, what to do?

Let's start at the beginning. I believe we can make one fundamental statement of fact. Everyone, especially *you,* wants the crew of your aircraft to be free of any medical deficiency that would interfere with safely and competently driving a flying machine from point A to point B. The pilot, however, wants this to be done without risking *himself* being booted out of flying for a living. There's the contradiction. But I can assure you that if the pilot does his part in learning the principles of health maintenance and how the FAA certifies him, there need not be the unnecessary threat that all pilots feel when their health is discussed or evaluated.

Pilots, like the rest of our structured society, rely heavily on rules and regulations, company policies, standards, SOP's, etc. to guide and direct us. If something does go wrong, we often can pass the buck to the rule maker or enforcer and thereby relieve ourselves of the responsibility. Not so with the pilot's health and medical certificate. The buck stops with the pilot!

Pilots already have a respected eduation in assuring that their airplanes meet mechanical and electronic criteria with the necessary help of specialists. In this regard, we have an enviable team. Yet, being human, we have a tendency to take short cuts or forget pertinent data in this complex profession, which is why we have checklists and proficiency checks. Also, as in any field of work, someone periodically has to check up on, or monitor, what we are doing. This is a fact of life in our society—no venture can meet the expectations of the people it services without some sort of monitoring. All of us need and silently expect someone to respectfully say, "Hey, what you're doing is OK," or "What you're doing *isn't* OK and you need to improve." This is true of pilots, as we all know. It is also true of business men and women, teachers, lawyers, and believe it or not, doctors.

How many times have you been to your private physician and felt you did not receive the best service that medicine could provide? As a doctor, I'm the first to say that you could, in fact, have been denied the best. Patients deserve the assurance of competent help, just as your passengers, expect you, unconditionally, to do your job safely—they expect a routine, uneventful flight each trip. What goes on behind that cockpit door is your business—as long as you do it right. To insure this, you must be monitored, even though you feel fine and *you* think you're healthy. Whose responsibility is this monitoring? Your peers protect you with professional standards and aeromedical committees. Your company protects you and its shareholders with check rides, company physicals and operating policies. And the FAA is supposed to protect the public from medically unsafe pilots through Federal Air Regulations and medical certification.

With the FAA's involvement in this monitoring process a multitude of things can happen—which is why these three letters, FAA, conjure up visions of a many-headed monster armed with a protocol on how to shaft the aviator at every turn. However, it is pertinent to understand the FAA's health monitoring philosophy and realize what *you* can do to keep the bureaucratic monster happy.

Let's review what I've stated so far:

1. The responsible pilot does not want to fly if he *knows* his health is going to interfere with his flying ability or potentially cause a disaster—and he certainly doesn't want anyone else flying in poor health.

2. There must be a monitoring program to protect, guide and assist the pilot and the pilot's peers, employer and passengers.

3. The FAA has been delegated as the government's agency to provide this monitoring program on behalf of the public.

But at this point, the process of insuring that only healthy pilots are flying often breaks down. Again, contrary to popular belief, the intent and objective of the FAA is not to ground pilots for insignificant medical reasons. The process will be discussed later, but for now let's make our first assumption.

Let's assume the FAA's sole *medical* goal is to assure that pilots do not have a medical problem that would create an unsafe situation. It's senseless to assume otherwise. (I am not discussing the age 60 rule.) It is also a fair assumption to recognize that most aircrews have little, if any, medical training, compared to the extent of their education in the equipment used in their profession—the aircraft, its components, and the environment in which they fly. It is indeed ironic and unfortunate that of the two most important parts of air travel, the pilot and his machine, the pilot is well educated only in the mechanics of his machine and not in the mechanics of himself—his health and his special maintenance requirements as a pilot. If some pilots treated their aircraft the way they treat their bodies, their aircraft would never reach its destination.

The military recognizes this need and quite effectively uses the "flight surgeon" system which requires that all flying personnel must see *only* a flight surgeon for *all* medical care—therapy, examination, general health, and certification of flying status. The flight surgeon is specifically trained in aviation medicine and devotes his full time to it, a fact that is generally recognized and respected by the aircrews. The result is trust and mutual understanding, and good medical care if the flight surgeon is doing his job. And the pilot is flying when he's healthy! The flight surgeon has the authority to return a pilot to flying status.

The military flight surgeon's civilian counterpart, the FAA-designated Aviation Medical Examiner, is not required to be specifically trained in aviation medicine beyond a three-day "familiarization course." An AME may devote most of his time to the practice of *non*-aviation medicine—family doctor, surgeon, internal medicine—and fit pilots in as his schedule permits. Just being a doctor does not assure knowledge of specific subject such as aviation medicine and aeromedical certification.

Another vitally important difference is that the military flight surgeon is considered to be a *part of the crew he serves*. He flies with, encounters delays with, eats questionable "meals" with, and suffers long days and short nights with the rest of the crew. The flight surgeon develops an acquaintance with the crew's peculiar physical and mental stresses, not to mention getting to know his pilot teammates individually. The crew also gets the chance to see just what the flight surgeon is up to and can "check him out," seeing whose side he's on. In the civilian aviation world, on the other hand, flying the jump seat is discouraged for even the most well-meaning AME.

To a certain extent the FAA attempts to follow the philosophy of the military flight-surgeon system. The Federal Air Surgeon in Washington has overall responsibility for aviation medicine and its consequences. The primary responsibility of *medical certification* is delegated to the FAA doctors in Oklahoma City. These doctors, in turn, have designated civilian physicians throughout the country to conduct the examinations *for* the FAA doctors. These local doctors, or AME's, have *no* authority except to certify healthy pilots—healthy as determined by the individual AME, but still subject to review by the FAA's doctors.

This process is why, for example, if your AME tells you that you have a "slight heart murmur" but *he* does not feel it is of any consequence, that AME has no authority to certify you without approval from the FAA Regional Flight Surgeon or the FAA physician in Oklahoma City. Sometimes, since the AME doesn't want to be the "bad guy," he may certify you, only to be reviewed (or monitored) later by the FAA. Weeks later, the FAA asks for more information and data from *you* to determine if the murmur is significant or potentially unsafe. The AME really could have done that to begin with, but for various reasons he chooses to let the FAA do the "dirty work." You're the one, however, whose career is on the line and, in your mind, now is being challenged.

Another policy of some AME's is to just not even check for any potential problems. It would appear that this "planned ignorance" keeps the pilots and the AME content, but those pilots sacrifice their health to protect their career—and often needlessly. Such "rubber stamping" AME's are around; worse, they often have a large following since they are the least threatening. In theory, this is the epitomy of irresponsibility, like ignoring a SIGMET or a thunderstorm simply because you have to get to your destination on time. But realistically, if in the same medical situation as a professional pilot, with my career at stake, I would be tempted to respond the same way. By ignoring potential problems, both the pilot and the doctor can plead innocent and make the FAA accept the responsibility. However, chances are the pilot will ultimately lose.

Although the FAA doctors often are made out to be the bad guys, they really aren't every time. The FAA, accept it or not, is no more a threat to your health and career than some AME's who *should* be acting in your best interests but, in fact, are not. Why? Why doesn't the FAA's program of pilot health monitoring work to the benefit of the pilot as well as the FAA?

An example may be in order. It is common knowledge that glaucoma is the leading cause of treatable progressive blindness after age 35. A doc pushing on your eyeballs with his fingers cannot rule out glaucoma unless it is far advanced. There is, however, a very simple test to check for the early presence of glaucoma by using an instrument called a tonometer. For reasons I cannot understand, many doctors doing allegedly complete "executive-type" physicals do not make this simple check. Many AME's follow the same routine, ignoring tonometry, while knowing full well that your vision is your most important human tool in flying. One of the reasons that the AME doesn't check it is because he hasn't done it before (or your new AME assumed that your other AME didn't do it). The pilot doesn't ask for it because he doesn't want any more information given to the FAA than necessary. Therefore, what was done (or not done) in previous exams plus the fear of knowing too much has established a precedent, one you don't want changed. The AME wants to be a "good guy," so he doesn't push the test on you. In fact, a well-meaning AME who does the simple test often is criticized for being "too thorough" and for jeopardizing the pilot's career; then the pilot probably will not return and will share his thoughts about that AME with other pilots. An AME is supposed to help you, but who is really helping whom?

Such "easy" physicians are more interested in having you return because of your acceptance than in preventing possible irreparable eye damage, despite the fact that the FAA will certify a pilot with glaucoma who is taking eye drops as long as his vision is *acceptable,* meaning it hasn't been destroyed too much by the delay in detection. A fair question is: If tonometry is so important, why doesn't the FAA require it? Well, the FAA knows that each doctor has different techniques; therefore, the FAA says that you can't have glaucoma or the effects of glaucoma, and lets your doctor determine whether or not you have glaucoma through his own methods. Thus, the monitor backs off and the doc gets by. Where do you stand? You could have early glaucoma, which is treatable and acceptable to the FAA, but you don't know it; then soon you begin to lose your vision and your career when it becomes noticeable to you. Where do you go now? To your AME? Your private doctor? The FAA?

One of the prime reasons for this breakdown is lack of adequate education and communication. You and I are trying to correct that. If you know why certain tests are done and what is at stake, you have a better control of your future. I will elaborate more in this book on the specific protocol that is followed, why it is essential, and how you can keep control. For now, I am stating that the greatest deterrent to the maintenance of your certification may be your peers and a few of the FAA's uninformed, inexperienced AME's who, by simply going through the motions and assuming they're doing you a favor, leave you holding the bag.

It is imperative that you be under the supervision of a physician who is knowledgeable in aviation medicine, FAA criteria, and the certification process. He must act as a military flight surgeon would act because his goal is to keep you flying safely. The doc must pursue the evaluation and certification process until a satisfactory result is achieved. That means, in addition to treating you in a manner acceptable to the FAA, he will coordinate, follow through, and personally insure that your certification is not compromised, that the medical data are accurate and complete, and that *you* are kept informed.

The aeromedical physician should guide you in how to keep healthy; to help you control your medical status. Together, you will monitor trends in the results of your exams and try to anticipate potential certification problems, resolving them before they interfere with your career. You should feel relatively comfortable in describing your aches, pains, and other complaints and be able to work together. After all, this doc should be a member of your team, as important to you as a mechanic or meteorologist.

Finding this perfect physician isn't all that easy, as we know. But until you do, there is a next-best thing: a health-maintenance program. In your situation, that also means an "FAA certification and career maintenance" program. Remember, your AME has little or no authority to keep you flying, *unless* you are truly healthy. The buck is still in your lap.

There are some things about your health that you can't control. You can't pick your parents, you can't alter your genes, and you can't change your potential for developing a disease not related to environment, such as cancer, vision changes and the aging process. In these situations, loss of license insurance and company benefits won't cure you or keep you flying.

But there are areas you can control, factors that, ignored or abused, invariably lead to deterioration of health that will affect only a *pilot's* career. With so much at stake—your career and love of flying—it would seem reasonable to expect that you would do everything possible to *maintain* your health, not waiting for a problem to get your attention. That means *preventive* maintenance just like the kind you provide the airplane in which you fly. Being grounded doesn't just happen to someone else. Your grounded buddy was feeling good too before he got the axe.

No one can do this work for you. No one can undo any permanent damage you have already allowed to occur, and no physician can do your health-maintenance work; indeed, physicians often can create more problems by letting you avoid this work.

Health Maintenance

You are quite capable of controlling the controllable elements of your health. Quit reading about the latest fad diets and physical conditioning programs in the scandal sheets and the popular lay magazines and books. They are not coming up with anything that is revolutionary. You wouldn't take flying lessons from them, so don't take their medical lessons either.

In brief, then:

1. You are in a profession that requires you to be free of disease that would interfere in the performance of your duties. "Feeling good" is not a true indicator of your health.

2. As in any other work, you must be monitored, and the FAA monitors you by using local AME's as their tools.

3. The process of medical certification through some local doctors with varying degrees of aeromedical knowledge, experience with the FAA, and interest in aviation, often leads to ignorance concerning your *actual* medical status. Consequently, your health is sacrificed for the sake of your career. It needn't be that way.

4. You are not concerned so much about being sick as you are about what happens when you are reported to the FAA

5. Finding a physician you can regard as a competent, respected "flight surgeon" is difficult. But you're stuck with having to see someone. All too often, pilots seek the doc that makes the fewest waves.

6. You will have the best chance of keeping certified if you program *yourself* to keep healthy, informed, and in top physical condition.

With the philosophy of pilot health monitoring and health maintenance in mind, let's look more closely at the medical standards the FAA expects you to meet.

2

Disqualifying Medical Conditions

A 36-year-old airline pilot was seeing his own family doctor on an annual basis in anticipation of his FAA exam. His family doctor noted his blood pressure had gone above 140/90, and as a result put him on a "new blood pressure medication." At his next FAA exam the blood pressure was still high, plus the pilot had to report that he was on medication. Three weeks later the FAA grounded him because of the hypertension and use of the blood pressure medication.

BASICALLY, THE FAA has fair medical criteria for certification of healthy pilots. In fact, if you were aware of the reasoning behind the FAA's medical decisions, you would probably agree with their conclusions in most cases challenged by pilots.

Now I'm sure that many of you are skeptical as you read this, especially if your opinion is based on your own experiences, those of your colleagues and your own interpretation of the FAA certification process. In defense, let me state clearly that I am in no way crusading for the FAA and its bureaucracy. I do believe, however, that the majority of *medical* decisions made about an individual pilot are fair, providing the FAA doctors have been given adequate documentation of that pilot's *true* medical status. I can appreciate your skepticism, but please bear with me and I hope you will understand why I have made such a controversial comment.

I would like to return to the analogy of the preventive maintenance program for your aircraft. There are tech orders, books on specifications, operation standards, ADs and a multitude of other complex, specific criteria that must be met during each periodic preventive maintenance inspection of the aircraft. Although the mechanic may simply sign off an aircraft and by so doing tells you that *he* feels everything is OK and the bird is airworthy and safe, you have the right — indeed, the responsibility — to check the records and the aircraft to insure that all of the specifications have, in fact, been met. You are not second-guessing or doubting the mechanic. In fact, most responsible mechanics are proud of their job and welcome the pilot's interest in their work. And you both speak the same "language" since, during your initial and recurrent training, you were and are educated as to how these specs were determined, why they are important and what restrictions must be met. In other words, *you* know what keeps your bird flying!

Meeting certain detailed "specifications" is no different when it comes to keeping your "human machines" out of trouble. Depending on whom you talk to, your body may be no more or less complex and difficult to handle and maintain than a complicated aircraft. To trust *only* a physician's simple statement that you are healthy enough to fly an airplane, rather than relying on a complete appraisal of "airworthiness," is not realistic. As I stated before, some physicians are not overly familiar with the medical standards necessary for a pilot, or the reasons for them, and the effect on a pilot's performance if they are not met. Therefore, the *medical* criteria that must be met by each pilot are documented in writing in the Federal Air Regulations, Part 67, and then further defined for the AME in the *"Guide for Aviation Medical Examiner's"* — both revised in the spring of 82. It should be accepted by us all that just as your aircraft needs *documented* specs to be met, your physiological and psychological specs necessary for safe flying, must also be documented so that you and others can be assured they have, in fact, been met.

The medical specs have one characteristic in your favor: The majority of the medical criteria are guidelines for the doctors and the FAA to follow. There is no hard and fast rule regarding the *individual pilot*. This allows for flexibility in determining the ultimate medical outcome by your aeromedical physician and the FAA as they review each medical case on its own individual merits. They then pass judgment, medically speaking, only on the individual pilot's ability to be a safe pilot *while flying*. You need not be in perfect health — just medically safe. For example, there are published acceptable limits for blood pressure. No pilot is judged by the FAA as having "hypertension" until he is fully evaluated and several blood pressure readings have been taken. However, if your AME doesn't provide the FAA with these data, and he submits just one *high* blood pressure reading (even though it is only slightly above the published maximums), there can be only one initial conclusion by the FAA — you have high blood pressure (or hypertension) until proven otherwise.

The FAA has one medical goal in defining the medical standards that all pilots must meet: To insure that each pilot is free of any medical problem that would interfere with the safe performance of his duties while flying. The U.S. Air Force differs in its regulations in that it spells out potential medical deficiencies far more elaborately than does the FAA. This is appropriate for the USAF flight surgeon system since the flight surgeon has more authority than the AME and there must be no doubt that each USAF pilot throughout the world is being adequately evaluated and meets strict, well-defined criteria. It used to be that the USAF medically certified its pilots of all its aircraft—all or none. The FAA, on the other hand, could functionally limit the operations of an aircraft on the medical and thus allow some pilots to fly with a medical problem but only in certain crew positions. However, this has now been reversed. The USAF now medically qualifies pilots for specific aircraft whereas the FAA has been instructed by the courts that it cannot limit functional operations for first class medicals. The new amendment, however, allows for functional limitations for second and third class medicals.

In my opinion, the keys to the FAA's medical certification policy are Federal Air Regulation (FAR) 61.53 which reads:

OPERATIONS DURING MEDICAL DEFICIENCY:

NO PERSON MAY ACT AS PILOT IN COMMAND, OR IN ANY OTHER CAPACITY AS A REQUIRED PILOT FLIGHT CREW MEMBER WHILE HE HAS A KNOWN MEDICAL DEFICIENCY, OR INCREASE OF A KNOWN MEDICAL DEFICIENCY THAT WOULD MAKE HIM UNABLE TO MEET THE REQUIREMENTS FOR HIS CURRENT MEDICAL CERTIFICATE.

and FAR 91.11(a)(3):

NO PERSON MAY ACT AS A CREWMEMBER OF A CIVIL AIRCRAFT WHILE USING ANY DRUG THAT AFFECTS HIS FACULTIES IN ANY WAY CONTRARY TO SAFETY.

Basically, these regulations mean that the decision to fly as a safe pilot is on *your* shoulders. They assume that you will accept the responsibility of being in good health and "ground" yourself should you develop a medical disability. The problem, of course, is: Do *you know* if you have a medical deficiency and whether it affects your flying? Your medical education in flight training, ground school and recurrent training is minimal at best. How are you expected to know if that pain in your chest is significant or why you can't fly with high blood pressure?

Keep in mind that you have the right to fly at any time while you carry a valid medical certificate, provided you can comply with FAR 61.53 and FAR 91.11(a)(3). In fact, look on the back of your medical certificate. You'll see a clear reminder to consider FAR 61.53 as part of *your* responsibility to be healthy while you are a crew member! Also keep in mind that this is Part *61* which applies to pilots, as apposed to

Disqualifying Medical Conditions

Part *67,* the medical criteria used by doctors. You could look at this as meaning that Part 67 is used to assist in the interpretation of the requirements that must be met in Part 61.53.

There is nothing mysterious about the content of Part 67 of the FARs. However, I have seen a variety of interpretations by attorneys, physicians, pilots and other "authorities," many of which are misleading or incomplete — and most of which leave you with more questions unanswered than answered, assuming you knew what questions to ask in the first place! Once again, let me state that there is a *medical* reason for every one of these medical regulations or standards but they are intended for use by doctors, not pilots, although they obviously have a direct effect on you. The legal interpretation is a matter for the courts and the NTSB.

When going through these regulations, it is important for you to realize that except for nine well-defined, specific medical disorders, the regulations are vague — for a reason: This allows the FAA to judge your medical problem on an individual basis and to interpret all available medical data, thus allowing reconsiderations, waivers and limitations, even though your health may not meet the letter of the law. Compare this to Part 121, which is rarely waived (the age 60 retirement rule is under Part 121 and therefore is not waiverable).

Part 67 basically defines the medical standards that must be met for First, Second and Third Class medical certificates. The protocol is the same for each level, but the range of acceptable limits differs. In other words, the exam should be the same for every pilot for any class — the *limits* you must meet depend on the class for which you are applying. The medical criteria as they pretain to a First-Class certificate are listed in paragraph 67.13, which I will discuss here, the Second and the Third-class requirements being less stringent variations of the same basic criteria.

Before we go into the regulations that govern the more common but less serious medical deficiencies, let's discuss the medical conditions where certificate denial is *mandatory* by the Aviation Medical Examiner. These are listed separately here since they pose the greatest threat to a pilot's career. The remainder of FAR 67 will be itemized in the appendix, with an explanation of each. I encourage you to scan the appendix to be familiar with its contents.

The majority of the medical disorders described relate to the *current* status of the disorder. That is, if you have a broken leg, you can't fly while it is healing; but once is has healed, there is no problem with flying. It's a different story for the "mandatory" disorders. It is important to note that these regulations state that even an established medical HISTORY of any of the nine conditions means a *mandatory* initial denial by the AME. For example, if you had a heart attack *twenty years ago* which has since completely resolved, a mandatory denial would still be required. As we will see, this mandatory denial by the AME sets the stage for further evaluation and collection of data to allow the FAA (not the AME) to judge whether or not you are safe to fly. Most of the reasoning behind denying certification to a pilot with a history of any one of the nine disorders should be self-explanatory, but the relationship of the *severity* of the disorder and its effect on your safe flying ability is often misunderstood. Therefore, I will take each one individually and attempt to clarify the justification for the *initial* denial. The following interpretations are my own and do not necessarily represent those of the FAA.

Conditions for Which Certificate Denial is Mandatory (Each of these disorders is clearly defined as a distinct FAR.)

I. A CHARACTER OR BEHAVIOR DISORDER WHICH IS SEVERE ENOUGH TO HAVE REPEATEDLY MANIFESTED ITSELF BY OVERT ACTS [FAR 67.13 (d)(1)(i)(a)]

We all know people who, in our own judgment, do strange things at strange times. This does not necessarily mean that the individual is mentally ill or that he has a severe mental disease requiring medication and psychiatric therapy. Overt means observable and not concealed. In other words, if a pilot has a disorder in his personality that could interfere with the performance of his duty as a crew member and he has shown he's not able to control himself in situations requiring his full attention, these outbursts would be considered "overt acts" that could reappear at inopportune times. Obviously this is a tough regulation to define, quantify and apply to an individual pilot, and is difficult to evaluate and document. It calls for subjective judgment and clear proof that the disorder would compromise safe flying. For example, if a pilot is afraid to fly in bad weather or is outwardly antagonistic towards many company policies, the presence of one of these "traits" is not in itself unsafe; but in situations of bad weather or maintaining morale on the flight deck, the results could be disastrous. Where is the "unsafe" point? Who should establish that point?

An additional part of the FAR states that a pilot can have no other personality disorder, neurosis or mental condition that the *Federal Air Surgeon* determines would make the applicant unable to safely perform the duties or exercise the privileges of the airman's medical certificate that he holds or for which he is applying. This is a "blanket" type regulation that covers any unsafe personality disorder not spelled out earlier.

Disqualifying Medical Conditions

II. A PSYCHOTIC DISORDER [FAR 67.13 (d)(1)(i)(b)]

Medically speaking, someone who is psychotic is definitely mentally ill. There are many types of psychotic disorders, with names you've heard like "split personality" or "paranoid" and "schizophrenic." These disorders are characterized by withdrawal from reality and an inability to cope with the usual stresses of life, certainly not those of a pilot. Psychoses usually require treatment which may include hospitalization, medication, and continuous psychiatric therapy. It is not difficult for a psychiatrist to diagnose and document a pilot who is clearly psychotic. There is often, however, poor acceptance of this diagnosis by the sick pilot and his peers, for there is much skepticism in the pilot community concerning psychiatry and psychology. I doubt, however, that any responsible pilot would allow a clearly *psychotic* pilot to fly either as a crew member or by himself.

III. CHRONIC ALCOHOLISM [FAR 67.13 (d)(1)(i)(c)]

This subject has been drawing a lot of attention in recent years, resulting in marked changes in the FAA's consideration for re-certifying rehabilitated alcoholics. It used to be that someone with a *history* of being an alcoholic, even if it was 25 years ago, could never fly again. Now, however, thanks to the combined efforts of ALPA and the FAA, after adequate therapy, "tincture of time," and documentation of sobriety along with an ongoing surveillance program, the FAA will consider certifying a pilot. The problem, of course, is in identifying and diagnosing a pilot as truly being a "chronic" alcoholic. The medical and mental professions are learning more about how to define a pilot who actually *is* an alcoholic, or how to determine whether he is a heavy social drinker or frequent abuser of alcohol. Alcoholism is chronic. It is a disease. The recent amendment now states: "—unless there is established clinical evidence, satisfactory to the Federal Air Surgeon, of recovery, including sustained total abstinence from alcohol for not less than the preceding 2 years". This allows for certification without an exemption. The 2 years period can also be reconsidered thru FAR 67.19 "Special Issue" and a recovered alcoholic can be returned to flying much sooner.

IV. DRUG ADDICTION (or drug dependence) [FAR 67.13 (d)(1)(i)(d)]

According to this regulation, addiction is a condition in which a person "is *dependent* on drugs other than alcohol, tobacco or caffeine-containing beverages, as evidenced by habitual use or clear sense of *need* for the drug." This is straightforward since, if you will recall, FAR 91.11 says *no* drugs of *any* kind may be used which could affect one's ability to fly. Although this usually implies narcotics, this also could mean any drug, even nonprescription over-the-counter medications. Even though we may be able to tolerate a specific drug at *ground* level environments, the effects of that drug can change dramatically at altitude, under stress, or both. Here again, I do not think too many responsible pilots would want someone as a crew member who could not function *without* drugs.

V. EPILEPSY (A convulsion or seizure disorder which can recur at any *unexpected* time) [FAR 67.13 (d)(2)(i)(a)]

The dilemma with this regulation is the *history* of epilepsy being disqualifying. That means, for example, if you had a convulsion even as a child, such as a "fever convulsion," this is technically disqualifying until proven completely resolved. What is difficult to determine is whether or not an individual who has epilepsy is, in fact, *controlled,* with or without medication. Medically speaking, a person who has had a convulsive attack of any kind has a greater chance of having another one at any time. Obviously, if medication is required to control the epilepsy, this use of drugs is also disqualifying.

VI. DISTURBANCE OF CONSCIOUSNESS WITHOUT SATISFACTORY EXPLANATION OF THE CAUSE [FAR 67.13 (d)(2)(i)(b)]

This includes that "mild concussion" you had back in high school as a football player. Pilots who have the potential for losing consciousness are obviously not qualified to be crew members. A physician cannot guarantee, unless all tests indicate otherwise, that an individual who has had any kind of disturbance of consciousness in the past will not have another occurrence. Unfortunately, medical science does not always come up with a specific answer to why a pilot has a disturbance of consciousness. Doctors can say what you *don't* have but may not be able to say what you *do* have. Therefore, you are left with a problem with no *known* cause or explanation! To almost anyone other than a pilot, this would not be a problem. In your case, passage of time, often years, is necessary before a doctor can reconsider the chances of a recurrence. However, *if,* as in a history of "mild concussion," the neurological evaluation is normal *and there is a satisfactory explanation which proves its insignificance,* the FAA usually will consider the application favorably.

VII. MYOCARDIAL INFARCTION (heart attack) [FAR 67.13 (e)(1)(i)]

This is straightforward, but often misunderstood. Why can't

Disqualifying Medical Conditions

a man fly simply because he had a heart attack five years ago — especially when he is in *better* shape and *better* health *now* than he ever was? The reason is that, statistically speaking, that pilot still has a greater chance of a recurrence than a pilot who has not had a heart attack, especially at altitude, even if the medical risk factors (hypertension, smoking, elevated cholesterol, etc.) have been *decreased* for that pilot. This will be discussed later. The FAA, however, is reconsidering a pilot's application with a heart attack history for medical certificates other than for First Class after passage of several years. As the state of the art of medical practice improves, even first class medicals will be issued. Another problem is that in some cases patients have been misdiagnosed as having had a heart attack when, in fact, it was some other medical problem, such as a pericarditis or a variation on an EKG or other test. Therefore, if a pilot has a *history* of a heart attack, this is disqualifying until it can be *proven* he has had no residual disease, that he has no current problems with his heart or coronary arteries, and has no cardiac factors.

As a part of the medical evaluation, for a first class medical certificate the FAA requires an EKG at certain ages. It is first required at age 35, then annually from age 40 on. One of the reasons for this is to show the absence of a previous undetected heart attack.

VIII. ANGINA PECTORIS OR CORONARY HEART DISEASE THAT HAS REQUIRED TREATMENT OR, IF UNTREATED, THAT HAS BEEN SYMPTOMATIC OR CLINICALLY SIGNIFICANT. [FAR 67.13 (e)(1)(ii)]

This regulation covers a multitude of potential problems. The key here is the *evidence* of disease in one or more of the coronary arteries (arteries that carry blood to the heart muscle itself). The only way this can be *dis*proven is with an angiogram (an x-ray of the coronary arteries) which is not usually recommended by your doctor as a routine test. There are now evaluations called the "thalium scan", "cat scan", etc, which are less of a risk but still expensive. And they are *not* conclusive. The presence of coronary artery disease is serious and is sometimes manifested by severe and disabling chest pain called "angina," which occurs when the heart muscle is not receiving an adequate supply of oxygen necessary to function properly. Therefore, in a physically demanding situation, when the heart is required to work even harder, it may fail, especially in hypoxic conditions.

A dilemma develops, for example, when a pilot has high blood pressure for any number of reasons and the FAA therefore requires a complete cardiovascular evaluation. As a part of this evaluation, an exercise cardiac stress test is necessary. As a result of this stress test, there could be a "suggestion" of coronary artery disease. Now the pilot faces *two* possible disqualifying conditions: high blood pressure and the stress-test abnormality—*which could be a normal variation*. This topic will be more fully discussed later; suffice it to say for now that coronary artery disease is a bona fide risk factor if *actually present*.

IX. DIABETES REQUIRING INSULIN OR ORAL HYPOGLYCEMICS]FAR 67.13 (f)(1)]

Diabetes is a disease that is poorly understood even by the medical profession. This is another topic that will be discussed later. The FAA assumes that the pilot's physician who makes the diagnosis of diabetes and prescribes drugs for it is sure of that diagnosis, has tried all other means to control it, and is left with insulin or oral hypoglycemics ("oral insulin") to control the diabetes. This is a sad situation for the inherently healthy pilot since the diabetes more than likely is the "mature onset" type, which means it has developed in the later years because of poor diet and physical conditioning. The diabetes can't be ignored and requires therapy, but it is probably directly related to that pilot's poor habits. Once he has diabetes, the burden is on the pilot to prove that it can be controlled through diet alone without medication—which he should have done in the first place.

A comment about the use of medication is in order. If a pilot requires medication to control a medical disorder, then it must be assumed that other measures have been tried and failed, such as diet, avoiding abuses, etc. In other words, it's not the side effects of the medication alone that are disqualifying; it is the fact that you have a disorder severe enough to require the *use* of the medicine.

When an Aviation Medical Examiner detects any of the nine disorders just described, he is required to deny the pilot's application for certification and to submit the information to the FAA.

However, keep this in mind: FAR 61.53 can also be interpreted to mean that if you are *not flying* with a known medical deficiency you are not breaking any regulations. Therefore, if you know you have a medical problem and are not flying but do not report it, nothing illegal is being committed. But, trying to hide any of these disorders and continuing to fly is a serious breach of responsibility and is illegal. The FAA wants AMEs to report *all* medical problems to keep a few irresponsible sick pilots from flying.

A key point to remember is that if you are healthy nobody really cares, especially the FAA. You will note that many of the criteria do

Disqualifying Medical Conditions

state that you must be *free* of that medical disorder but they don't say that you have to be healthy. They mean the same thing, but because of the wording, it would appear that the AME and the FAA have a negative approach, as if they are *only* looking for something wrong (and consequently are "out to get you"). They are, but only in the sense of proving the absence of a medical problem that would interfere with your safe flying. If nothing can be found, then usually nothing is said.

We have considered the nine most important medical standards that *must* be met. The rest of Part 67 as to pertains to the First Class medical certificate will be found in the Appendix. Keep in mind that some of these will be numerical standards that must be met, such as blood pressure, vision, hearing, and so on. Whereas, in other cases, meeting the standards of the absence of disease will be proof that you do not have any specific medical problems. Remember, basically the medical FARs are realistic and fair—if used correctly by your doctor and your AME.

What we have discussed thus far are the specific *regulations* which deal with medical standards. Except for the nine designated medical problems requiring denial by the AME yet still certifiable by the Federal Air Surgeon, the rest of these FARs are not specific, that is, they are expressed in general terms. The AME therefore uses a manual entitled *Guide for Aviation Medical Examiners,** published by the FAA to assist the doctor in complying with the FARs. This publication lists some of the specific medical disorders that would deny or defer certification.

Once again, keep in mind that although the healthy pilot gets little recognition, the healthy pilot is the only pilot an AME can certify. In essence, the medical examiner is evaluating the applicant to prove the *absence* of any medical disorder that would create a hazard to flying. The AME can *defer* the issuance of the certificate, which means that although an applicant may have a medical problem, he is not necessarily *permanently* grounded although the pilot can't fly now. Once he's been deferred or reported to the FAA, additional information from tests not normally a part of the usual FAA exam must be completed and reviewed by the FAA before the applicant can be certified. The medical examiner, therefore, has *only* the responsibility of proving during his examination that the *applicant does not have* any of the medical disqualifications noted in the guide. If he has a potentially disqualifying medical problem, only the FAA can certify him.

Appendix II has a complete listing of the different specific items that must be evaluated and commented on by the medical examiner.

---

*The FAA has recently revised the guide and it is in the hands of most AME's. The last revision was in 1970!

The items listed follow the same format as on the FAA Form 8500-8 (your application for medical certification). The listed items cannot be considered a comprehensive tabulation of all the possible medical disorders that would interfere with flying safely, nor is the list one which is cast in concrete when considering you as being safe to fly. That is, many of the listed conditions can be certified after an adequate evaluation and review by the FAA.

You may want to defer reading the Appendix unless a specific disorder or medical condition interests you. For now, it is important to remember that this partial list is what you are judged by. You must be able to meet the standard *every time you fly*. Since you can't take a physical every day, *you* must play doctor and decide if you are safe to fly (we are back to FAR 61.53 which says you can't fly with a known medical disorder).

Another important point is that the burden really is on you, not the AME, to further elaborate a medical disorder. In other words, the FAA corresponds with you, not the AME. The reason is that you have the choice of seeing which ever doctor you want. The examiner can help and coordinate the evaluation and make the whole process more efficient for you, but it's still your problem.

One final item of Form 8500-8 is that section filled out by the examiner—Item 61, COMMENTS ON HISTORY AND FINDINGS: RECOMMENDATIONS. This is an area where Aviation Medical Examiners could forego many delays in the certification process; if they would just take the time to explain an abnormality found on the evaluation or supplement the data with other tests or visits to specialists, a lot of time and confusion could be saved. The pilot applicant would not be sitting around wondering what is going to happen with the FAA. However, it is much easier for some examiners to simply submit brief medical data to the FAA and then let the FAA be the one to ask you for more data, come up with the conclusion, and be the "bad guy." This could be avoided in many cases simply with the examiner's explanation and providing the expected additional information for the FAA.

The combination of the medical history checked off by the pilot applicant on the front of the FAA Form 8500-8 and the examination report by the examiner on the back constitute the information sent to the FAA. If everything fits into the proper criteria and all the blanks are filled in, the local examiner can certify. However, he has no authority to certify if the applicant does not meet these criteria until further evidence is provided and approved by the FAA.

Keep in mind that the standards, criteria, and guidelines are used to determine if you are qualified to fly from day to day just as if you were asked to pass your physical every day prior to your trip. The key, once again, is FAR 61.53. If you are healthy—OK—go flying. If you're not healthy, then what? Any medical disability is subject to interpretation by your doctor, your AME, and the FAA. If there is no potential problem in regard to your flying responsibility, there is no reason why you cannot be certified.

Although the letter of the law has not changed until recently (and that change, was mainly administrative), the significance of the status of your health to flying has changed. Every condition is subject to interpretation, and the Federal Air Surgeon has the authority and flexibility to make judgement decisions. If you are safe to fly based on *current* medical experience and interpretation, he can certify you. This is why it is vitally important that those who sit in judgment be provided with as much pertinent information as possible to enable them to reach a responsible conclusion. Inadequate or incomplete reports will be looked upon as simply that. The FAA will return a judgment, saying "based on the information received" and will state its conclusion.

We've all heard "war stories" from friends and peers who would dispute my original comment that the medical criteria of the FAA are fair. However, if the full truth were known about the circumstances in each case, one actually would find that inadequate information was supplied or that the applicant was not really aware of the significance of the disorder and did not understand its implications for safe flying. These "war stories" are not valid scientific data and the pilot's peers should not pass judgment on a certain individual's medical problem and his flying status until all the facts are known. More than likely, that "sick" pilot judged OK by his "lay" peers should, in reality, not be flying.

My sole purpose for reminding you of this is not to justify the FAA's actions, but rather to encourage you to disregard what you hear in the rumor mill and pursue evaluation of a medical disorder either known or suspected, with competent aeromedical physicians who are aware of FAA protocol and requirements and who will personally assist you in acquiring the necessary documentation to justify your certification **before** making reports to the FAA.

You will note that the regulations and the *Guide* specify that the *applicant* is the one who is responsible for resolving a medical disorder. The point is that you, the pilot, must know where you truly stand medically and what your options are in terms of your required evaluation. It is up to *you* to insure that any disorder that has been found is expeditiously and efficiently handled.

There are key points throughout the chapter that you must remember. The following is a review of those that will keep you flying and help you understand what's at stake.

Pilot's Manual of Medical Certification

Key Points

1. All of the disqualifying disorders can interfere with safe flying.
2. The added risk of a possible recurrence of those disorders often complicates the final judgment.
3. Simply because there are no symptoms doesn't mean you are not a potential risk or don't have a problem. It is up to the AME and the FAA to insure that no problem exists.
4. In the *absence* of a disorder that *would* be hazardous to flying, and with adequate valid data, you *can* fly—you need not be in perfect health.
5. If you suspect you have a problem or you bust a physical, no report need be made to the FAA—if you don't fly.
6. When you can prove your good health, *then* the report is submitted to the FAA, and if you are healthy, it will certify you.
7. The FAA corresponds with you, the pilot—not the AME—for any additional workup. Therefore, *you* are responsible for maintaining your flying status.
8. A dismissal is not final. You can always be reconsidered.

3

The FAA's Certification Process

A 40-year-old corporate pilot had seen the same AME for years without any mention of problems. However, this time his AME was not available and he saw another AME who was more thorough and detected a murmur. This doctor stated that the murmur was not significant, but the doctor also admitted that he wasn't familiar with what the FAA wanted; consequently, he did not certify the pilot and submitted the data to the FAA. The pilot was grounded, didn't know where to go, and had to wait four weeks to hear from the FAA. Eventually, after four months of seeing specialists and sending in reports, he was back flying. The murmur couldn't be ignored, but the pilot need not have been grounded for five months.

FLYING IS ALMOST A SIXTH SENSE to you. You're a good "stick and rudder" pilot. In fact, you rarely have to think about what you are doing with your hands and feet as you "drive" your machine down the ILS. Remember way back when you began flying? It took a long time and a lot of practice and experience before you got this "straight and level" act together, and your steep turns were anything but coordinated. While you are recalling those exciting days, consider this: How would you explain to me *in writing* the procedure for executing a coordinated standard-rate turn? It's very difficult since you can't expect me to understand what you are describing without my already knowing the basics of how to fly. The only way to be sure that I can comprehend what you are describing is to have me read your description *more than once*.

I want you to be as famliar with how you are medically certified as you are with the basic technique of flying. Consequently, I face a similar problem in describing the certification process. Next to the chapters on your own health-maintenance program, this chapter is probably the most important in keeping your certification. But I can't expect you to comprehend what I am describing without assuming that you already know about part of this certification process. To be sure

29

that I keep this subject clear in your mind, I will add my personal comments to the description of the actual protocol of the certification process.

We established that a monitoring program is necessary to insure that only healthy pilots control aircraft. The FAA has this responsibility and as a result has developed a list of medical conditions potentially incompatible with safe flying. This chapter will describe how you are medically evaluated to determine the presence or absence of these conditions, and the administrative sequence of the certification process, including reconsiderations and appeals if you fail the physical.

THE CERTIFICATION PROCESS IN GENERAL
The Medical Application and Examination

You must go to a designated FAA medical examiner—the AME of your choice—for the FAA physical. This AME is a physician designated by the FAA to provide the medical data with which the FAA can pass judgment. When you arrive for each FAA exam, you are, in effect, applying *anew,* as if this were the first time. The FAA Form 8500-8 (Application for Airman Medical Certificate) is actually an *application* to the FAA for a medical certificate. Obviously, past applications are considered in the final analysis by the FAA, but at the time you are in the AME's office, you are essentially *re-*applying. If all is OK, you are asking the FAA to certify you as being healthy based on this medical information, and your AME has the authority to certify you. If you are not OK, the AME does *not* have the authority to certify you unless the FAA has granted its approval.

Therefore, if there are no disqualifying conditions noted during your medical examination, you promptly are certified for the period of your medical classification (First Class is for six months, Second is for twelve months, Third is for twenty-four months). Most pilots do not think much about their medical status in the interim and do little to prepare themselves for the *next* FAA exam. Keep in mind that although you have a current medical certificate in your pocket, you remain subject to FAR 61.53—namely that you can't fly with a known medical problem. Regardless of when you passed your last physical, if *you* know that you are not healthy enough to fly, then you can't fly until your health is reviewed by the FAA or your AME. In other words, if you can't pass a flying physical on each day that you fly, then you can't legally or safely fly, even though you may have had a good physical two weeks before. Since you aren't a doctor, it is often difficult for you to determine what needs to be done when you're not feeling right. We'll discuss this predicament in detail later in this chapter.

If at your examination something is *not* OK, a whole new process will begin, either to confirm the justification to disqualify you or to determine that the medical condition is not, in fact, a deterrent to safe

The FAA's Certification Process

MEDICAL CERTIFICATE _____ CLASS AND STUDENT PILOT CERTIFICATE

THIS CERTIFIES THAT *(Full name and address)*

has met the medical standards prescribed in Part 67, Federal Aviation Regulations for this class of Medical Certificate.

DATE OF BIRTH	HEIGHT	WEIGHT	HAIR	EYES	SEX

LIMITATIONS

DATE OF EXAMINATION	EXAMINER'S SERIAL NO.

EXAMINER SIGNATURE

TYPED NAME

AIRMAN'S SIGNATURE

WHEN ISSUED AS A MEDICAL-STUDENT PILOT CERTIFICATE, the holder has met standards prescribed in Part 61, FAR's for such certificate, and is prohibited from carrying passengers.

TOTAL PILOT TIME	16. TO DATE	17. LAST 6 MOS.
CIVIL		
MILITARY		

APPLICATION FOR ☐ AIRMAN MEDICAL CERTIFICATE ☐ AIRMAN MEDICAL AND STUDENT PILOT CERTIFICATE

Please print these items

1. FULL NAME *(Last, first, middle)* | PATH CONTROL

2A. ADDRESS *(No. Street, City, State, ZIP No.)* | 2B. SOCIAL SECURITY No.

County:

2C. PLACE OF BIRTH *(Student pilot applicants only)*

3. DATE OF BIRTH *(Mo., day, year)*	4. HEIGHT *(Inches)*	5. WEIGHT *(Pounds)*	6. COLOR OF HAIR	7. COLOR OF EYES	8. SEX

9A. CLASS OF MEDICAL CERTIFICATE APPLIED FOR	9B. TYPE OF AIRMAN CERTIFICATE(S) HELD		
	AIRLINE TRANSPORT		FLIGHT INSTRUCTOR
FIRST	COMMERCIAL		PRIVATE
SECOND	ATC SPECIALIST		STUDENT
THIRD	FLIGHT ENGINEER		NONE
	FLIGHT NAVIGATOR		OTHER

10. OCCUPATION *(If ATC Specialist, specify position and facility)*

11. EXTENDED ACTIVE DUTY MEMBER OF		12. EMPLOYER
a. AIR FORCE	d. COAST GUARD	
b. ARMY	e. NATL. GUARD	13. LENGTH OF TIME IN PRESENT OCCUPATION
c. NAVY/MARINES	f. NONE	
MILITARY SERVICE NO.		14. PRIMARY TYPE OF FLYING
		BUSINESS / PLEASURE

15. CURRENTLY USE ANY MEDICATION *(Including eye drops)*
YES — TYPE AND PURPOSE
NO

18. HAS AN FAA AIRMAN MEDICAL CERTIFICATE EVER BEEN DENIED, SUSPENDED, OR REVOKED	19. HAVE YOU, AS A PILOT, HAD AN AIRCRAFT ACCIDENT WITHIN THE PAST 2 YEARS	20. DATE OF LAST FAA PHYSICAL EXAM *(If none, state so)*
YES DATE	YES DATE	
NO	NO	

21. MEDICAL HISTORY — HAVE YOU EVER HAD OR HAVE YOU NOW **ANY OF** THE FOLLOWING: *(For each "yes" checked, describe condition in REMARKS)*

Yes	No	Condition	Yes	No	Condition	Yes	No	Condition	Yes	No	Condition
		a. Frequent or severe headaches			g. Heart trouble			m. Nervous trouble of any sort			s. Medical rejection from or for military service
		b. Dizziness or fainting spells			h. High or low blood pressure			n. Any drug or narcotic habit			t. Rejection for life insurance
		c. Unconsciousness for any reason			i. Stomach trouble			o. Excessive drinking habit			u. Admission to hospital
		d. Eye trouble except glasses			j. Kidney stone or blood in urine			p. Attempted suicide			v. Record of traffic convictions
		e. Hay Fever			k. Sugar or albumin in urine			q. Motion sickness requiring drugs			w. Record of other convictions
		f. Asthma			l. Epilepsy or fits			r. Military medical discharge			x. Other illnesses

REMARKS *(If no changes since last report, so state)*

FOR FAA USE REVIEW ACTION CODES

22. HAVE YOU EVER BEEN ISSUED A STATEMENT OF DEMONSTRATED ABILITY (WAIVER)	NO	PHYSICAL DEFECTS NOTED ON STATEMENT OF DEMONSTRATED ABILITY (WAIVER)	WAIVER SERIAL NO.
	YES *(Give defects and waiver no.)*		

23. MEDICAL TREATMENT WITHIN PAST 5 YEARS

DATE	NAME AND ADDRESS OF PHYSICIAN CONSULTED	REASON

— NOTICE —
Whoever in any matter within the jurisdiction of any department or agency of the United States knowingly and willfully falsifies, conceals or covers up by any trick, scheme, or device a material fact, or who makes any false, fictitious or fraudulent statements or representations, or makes or uses any false writing or document knowing the same to contain any false, fictitious or fraudulent statement or entry, shall be fined not more than $10,000 or imprisoned not more than 5 years, or both. (U.S. Code, Title 18, Sec. 1001.)

24. APPLICANT'S DECLARATION
I hereby certify that all statements and answers provided by me in this examination form are complete and true to the best of my knowledge, and I agree that they are to be considered part of the basis for issuance of any FAA certificate to me. I have also read and understand the Privacy Act statement that accompanies this form.

SIGNATURE OF APPLICANT *(In ink)* | DATE

FAA FORM 8500-8 (10-75)   SUPERSEDES PREVIOUS EDITION   Form Approved. OMB No. 04-R0089

Pilot's Manual of Medical Certification

REPORT OF MEDICAL EXAMINATION

NOR-MAL	CHECK EACH ITEM IN APPROPRIATE COLUMN (Enter NE if not evaluated)	AB-NOR-MAL	NOTES: Describe every abnormality in detail, enter applicable item number before each comment. Use additional sheets if necessary and attach to this form.
	25. Head, face, neck and scalp		
	26. Nose		
	27. Sinuses		
	28. Mouth and throat		
	29. Ears, general *(Internal and external canals) (Auditory acuity under item 49)*		
	30. Drums *(Perforation)*		
	31. Eyes, general *(Visual acuity under items 50 & 51)*		
	32. Ophthalmoscopic		
	33. Pupils *(Equality and reaction)*		
	34. Ocular motility *(Associated parallel movement, nystagmus)*		
	35. Lungs and chest *(Including breasts)*		
	36. Heart *(Thrust, size, rhythm, sounds)*		
	37. Vascular system		
	38. Abdomen and viscera *(Including hernia)*		
	39. Anus and rectum *(Hemorrhoids, fistula, prostate)*		
	40. Endocrine system		
	41. G—U system		
	42. Upper and lower extremities *(Strength, range of motion)*		
	43. Spine, other musculoskeletal		
	44. Identifying body marks, scars, tattoos		
	45. Skin and lymphatics		
	46. Neurologic *(Tendon reflexes, equilibrium, senses, coordination, etc.)*		
	47. Psychiatric *(Specify any personality deviation)*		FOR FAA USE - PATHOLOGY CODE NOS.
	48. General systemic		

49. HEARING — RIGHT EAR | LEFT EAR | **50. DISTANT VISION** *(Standard test types only)* | **51. NEAR VISION** *(Use linear values)*

WHISPERED VOICE (STANDING SIDEWAYS DISTANT EAR CLOSED) ___ FT. ___ FT.
AUDIOMETER *(Decibel Loss)* 500 1000 2000 4000 500 1000 2000 4000

	RIGHT EYE	20/	CORRECTED TO 20/	20/	CORRECTED TO 20/
	LEFT EYE	20/	CORRECTED TO 20/	20/	CORRECTED TO 20/
	BOTH EYES	20/	CORRECTED TO 20/	20/	CORRECTED TO 20/

52. INTRAOCULAR TENSION *(Tonometry required for Air Traffic Control Specialist)*

	RIGHT EYE	LEFT EYE
TACTILE		
TONOMETRIC		

53. COLOR VISION *(Test used, number of plates missed)*

54. FIELD OF VISION | **55. HETEROPHORIA DIOPTERS** *(Not required for Class Three)*

RIGHT EYE | LEFT EYE | DISTANCE | ESOPHORIA | EXOPHORIA | RIGHT H. | LEFT H.

56. BLOOD PRESSURE | **57. PULSE** *(Wrist)*

RECUMBENT, MM MERCURY | SYSTOLIC | DIASTOLIC | RESTING | AFTER EXERCISE | 2 MINUTES AFTER EXERCISE

58. URINALYSIS | **59. ECG** *(Date)* | **60. OTHER TESTS**

ALBUMIN | SUGAR

61. COMMENTS ON HISTORY AND FINDINGS; RECOMMENDATIONS *(Attach all consultation reports, ECGs, X-rays, etc. to this report before mailing)*

FOR FAA USE
CODED
PUNCHED
VERIFIED

62. APPLICANT'S NAME | **63. DISQUALIFYING DEFECTS** *(List by item no.)*

EXAMINER CODES

HAS BEEN ISSUED ☐ MED. CERTIF. ☐ MED. AND STUDENT PILOT CERTIF.
NO CERTIF. ISSUED - FURTHER EVALUATION REQUIRED
HAS BEEN DENIED - LETTER OF DENIAL ISSUED (Copy attached)

CLERICAL REJECT

64. MEDICAL EXAMINER'S DECLARATION — *I hereby certify that I personally examined the applicant named on this medical examination report, and that this report with any attachment embodies my findings completely and correctly.*

DATE OF EXAMINATION | AVIATION MEDICAL EXAMINER'S NAME AND ADDRESS (Type or print) | AVIATION MEDICAL EXAMINER'S SIGNATURE flying. Suppose that a medical problem is detected, even though you haven't noticed any symptoms and you didn't have the problem the last time you took the physical. The FAA will want more information. An important point to remember at this state is that, unless your AME anticipates what the FAA needs, the FAA will correspond with *you*, not the AME, on what the FAA needs.

The FAA's Response to the Application

All applications, regardless of the results, are sent to the Aeromedical Certification Branch of the FAA in Oklahoma City. This office receives about 2,200 applications per day! Results of each application must be fed into the computer before any action is taken, a process which takes about two to three weeks. Any abnormal, incomplete or equivocal application which suggests you aren't fit to fly has to be reviewed by a doctor, not the computer. The FAA doctor does not get the opportunity to pass judgment on an application until several weeks have passed from the time it was mailed from your AME's office. Futhermore, sitting on the doc's desk are many applications that arrived before yours. It is no wonder there are delays in the certification process. Remember, you may know you have a problem and don't have a certificate with which to fly, but you must wait for the FAA to respond to your application by writing to you before you can even begin to work towards getting your certificate back.

I would like to put in a few words for these "humans," the physicians and their assistants in this medical certification branch of the FAA as well as the other aeromedical offices of the FAA. Contrary to what many pilots think, these are caring people. They have no desire to "ground" you just for kicks. A grounded pilot means more work for the FAA, something they don't need since they tend to be chronically behind in their administrative objectives. They have an awesome responsibility to certify only those pilots who are not likely to get sick while flying. Many pilots, with their careers hanging in the balance, feel that the bureaucracy of the FAA is and historically has been impersonal, uncaring and downright unreasonable. This is not true of the *medical* personnel of the FAA. I know this because I have worked with these people and have seen them at work. They also must follow bureaucratic rules and work within difficult limitations. If given the *opportunity* to help the grounded pilot, the aeromedical certification people of the FAA will do their best to arrive at a fair yet responsible decision. Many pilots will not agree with my observation and have their own "war stories" to tell. However, if all the facts were known about those cases, I doubt that most would find the FAA solely to blame for results considered unfair. The FAA doctors are not always right about a pilot, but they seldom are wrong in their decisions *based on the data supplied to them!* This is an important distinction.

Another misconception is that a pilot's certificate may be "pulled" or taken away by the FAA while he is certified. Actually, this *only* happens when the FAA determines that the pilot has a disqualifying condition *after* the AME has certified him and has already given him the "ticket" (medical certificate). In most initial FAA exams by the AME, the certificate is simply not issued when a problem is noted, and the pilot cannot legally fly. This is a picky point, but this misunderstanding leads to increased fear of the FAA. The reason your ticket is "pulled" at a later date may not be the fault of the FAA. It may be that some AMEs fail to detect a problem later *identified* by the FAA when medical data are reported by the AME. The result, however, is the same: A grounded pilot. Your AME should have the guts to tell you when he knows that you don't pass or there is something suspicious instead of implying that everything was OK and forcing the FAA to "pull your ticket" later. If handled properly by the AME in the beginning, there is no need for the FAA to "pull your ticket" *after* you were misled into thinking that you were qualified.

Denied Examination/Applications

After the FAA *doctor* in Oklahoma City has dug down to your "abnormal, incomplete or equivocal" application and finds that it *possibly* is disqualifying, he replies directly to *you,* either by requesting additional information or confirming the AME's denial. If you are denied, this letter fully explains the appeal procedure to you. If more information is required and an appeal is suggested, a time limit is stated, such as 30, 60 or 90 days, depending on your medical condition and its effect on safe flying. The purpose of this is twofold: first to determine the amount of time your file is reasonably kept active and your certificate is kept valid by the FAA; and second, it is a technique to determine how serious you are in pursuing your medical certification. *Your file can be reopened at any time.* For example, if a letter states that you have 60 days to respond, and you don't, the FAA interprets this to mean either that you couldn't document that your medical condition was not disqualifying (and the FAA has no way of knowing this unless a report is sent to them), or that you are not interested in pursuing your certificate. After the deadline, you are no longer legally medically certified even if you had been certified by the AME. If you simply couldn't get the medical evaluation done before the deadline, you only have to submit the data to reopen your file and begin the appeal process again. You can call the FAA for an extension and explain why. If it is reasonable, they might agree and allow you to keep flying during your evaluation.

The Federal Air Surgeon in Washington, D. C., will pass judgment on certain more serious or complicated medical conditions that the Oklahoma City doctors or the Regional Flight Surgeons do not have authority to judge. He will use the expertise of other specialists. However, the vast majority of disqualifying conditions that can eventually be certified can be judged in Oklahoma City if enough information is given. This is an important point. *The FAA doctors, wherever they are located, cannot act in your best interests unless provided with adequate medical reports.* It would be like you making a weather decision based only on the temperature and wind velocity. There is no way you can justify your decision of going in adverse weather without more data. The FAA doctors have the same problem with your application and file.

THE CERTIFICATION PROCESS, IN DETAIL

Now that you have an overview of the process, let's go back to the beginning, to the point at which you walk into your AME's office, and more clearly explain the procedure. You can see any AME you choose, even a different one each time if you wish. Whether it is your first visit or the 20th, the *procedure* used to certify you should be the same. The *interpretation* of the same information obtained from the medical examination can differ from one AME to another—and often does. It is threatening enough to you to know this, but we also know that both the exam and the subsequent results will have as many variations as the number of doctors that you go to, even though the procedure of the certification process should be the same. For example, one AME may say you have an abnormal EKG. You, on your own, go to another AME and he says that the EKG poses no problem. Only the FAA, in the final analysis, has the authority to decide, providing it is given the right data. The more you know how the process works, the more control you have of keeping your application from being misjudged by the FAA.

The Application and the AME

You first fill out the front part of the FAA form 8500-8. This part is self-explanatory and is similar to any other medical history form, such as a standard insurance application. It could be tempting not to admit past or present conditions that you know will be disqualifying. I can't honestly disagree with the motivation, knowing that your career is at stake, and you no doubt have thought: "Who's to know as long as I feel OK?" But hiding even a small abnormality is unwise, because you could be, in fact, not only threatening your career but also your responsibility as a pilot by having a potentially dangerous medical condition while not being aware of it. Equally important, the odds are that the problem is resolvable. Also, on the FAA 8500-8 form you declare, in no uncertain terms, that you have answered the questions factually, to the best of *your* knowledge—and you sign your name to that fact. For your own sake, check again what you are signing as being

Pilot's Manual of Medical Certification

factual the next time you fill out the 8500-8. Remember, should there be *any* reason to review your medical files, such as after a minor incident while flying or worse, any *known* medical problem that you "overlooked" could be reason enough to end your career. The medical problem you were hiding could have been insignificant, but the fact that you deceived the FAA is enough to jeopardize your career.

The Examination

After filling out your portion of the 8500-8, you are now subjected to various tests and the physical exam.

Your vision should be tested by either reading a chart 20 feet away in a well-lighted area or by using an appropriate apparatus which, through the use of mirrors, duplicates the conditions of near and distant objects.

Your eyes should be checked for glaucoma, since there is nothing to be gained by ignoring the test; in fact, ignoring tonometry could lead to loss of your vision as well as your career. Obviously the test is desirable and totally to your advantage. The FAA will accept most glaucomas when treated by eye drops if your vision hasn't already deteriorated so much that you can't pass the visual acuity test.

An audiogram should always be performed. Using the whispered voice to determine hearing ability is grossly inaccurate. The object of a hearing test is to determine an unknown hearing loss *before* it becomes disqualifying. Corrective action may be taken to prevent further hearing loss and save your hearing as well as your career. Trying to "get by" by using the whispered voice is, in my opinion, foolish and similar in purpose to cramming for an exam just to get by, even though the material in the exam is important. Just "getting by" on hearing is really taking an unnecessary chance.

A urine specimen is tested for the presence of sugar, which could signify diabetes or the tendency toward it, and albumin, which might indicate kidney disease.

Your blood pressure and pulse are taken. Note that the FAA requests a "recumbent" blood pressure—blood pressure taken while lying down. This is the FAA's way of giving you the best chance of passing. More on these topics later.

The physical examination is done by the AME. Contrary to some opinions the *examination* should be the same for all classes of medical certification. The difference between First, Second and Third Class is in the stringency of the criteria that must be met (which may include a few extra tests) by each applicant pilot, not in the *type* of physical given. However, the AME may be as critical with his evaluation as he feels is necessary for the type of flying to be done. The more knowledgeable an AME is about flying and the bureaucracy of the FAA, the more that AME can be a true asset to you. An AME who is a "white knuckler" when it comes to flying could be overly critical. One who has no interest in flying or in working with the FAA may take the whole medical evaluation process for granted and not accept the importance of the exam. The pilot who knows he is in good health because he has had a complete "executive" type of physical by someone who may not be familiar with the FAA certification process or the effects of a problem on safe flying has an additional potential threat built into his career maintenance: a false sense of security. A single battery of blood tests does not prove you are in good health unless those results are considered along with the rest of an exam. Ideally, the AME should be a pilot himself and should be familiar with the requirements of FAA protocol and should desire to assist you in your certification beyond the initial medical exam.

The *Usual* Outcome of the Examination

After the exam, the AME reviews all the data obtained from your medical history, the testing procedures and his examination. He will then determine if you have any disqualifying conditions as defined in the AME's guide. If there are none noted, he will certify you. Basically, the AME need only obtain the minimum data, make a decision to certify or not certify, and submit the 8500-8 to the FAA for final judgment. The *FAA* then determines how appropriate it would be to issue your certificate with or without a waiver or limitation.

There is one situation that warrants comment: the disqualifying condition that is recognized by the AME, but for various reasons, he may not mention anything to the pilot. In this situation, the pilot leaves the office assuming that all is OK, only to get a letter several weeks or months later stating that there is, in fact, a potential abnormality requiring more data before the FAA can legally certify him. There are few situations that are more scary to a pilot than this! I feel there are few circumstances, if any, in which the AME cannot anticipate the FAA's response to his findings even before the 8500-8 is submitted to the FAA, and he can usually do whatever is necessary to assist the pilot in resolving the problem. However, the AME who elects to react by not telling you the whole story does so to maintain his reputation as a "good guy' to you and remain on your good side so that you will return to him for your next exam. No AME really wants to ground a pilot. So, this guy lets the FAA lay the bad news on you; indeed, the FAA encourages AMEs to do this in order to maintain the AME's respectability and the trust of the rest of the pilot group. The FAA assumes, though, that this AME has performed a good evaluation and has at least informed the pilot of what to expect, even if the doctor doesn't want to get involved. This preparation isn't always accom-

Pilot's Manual of Medical Certification

IMPROPERLY MANAGED CERTIFICATION SEQUENCE

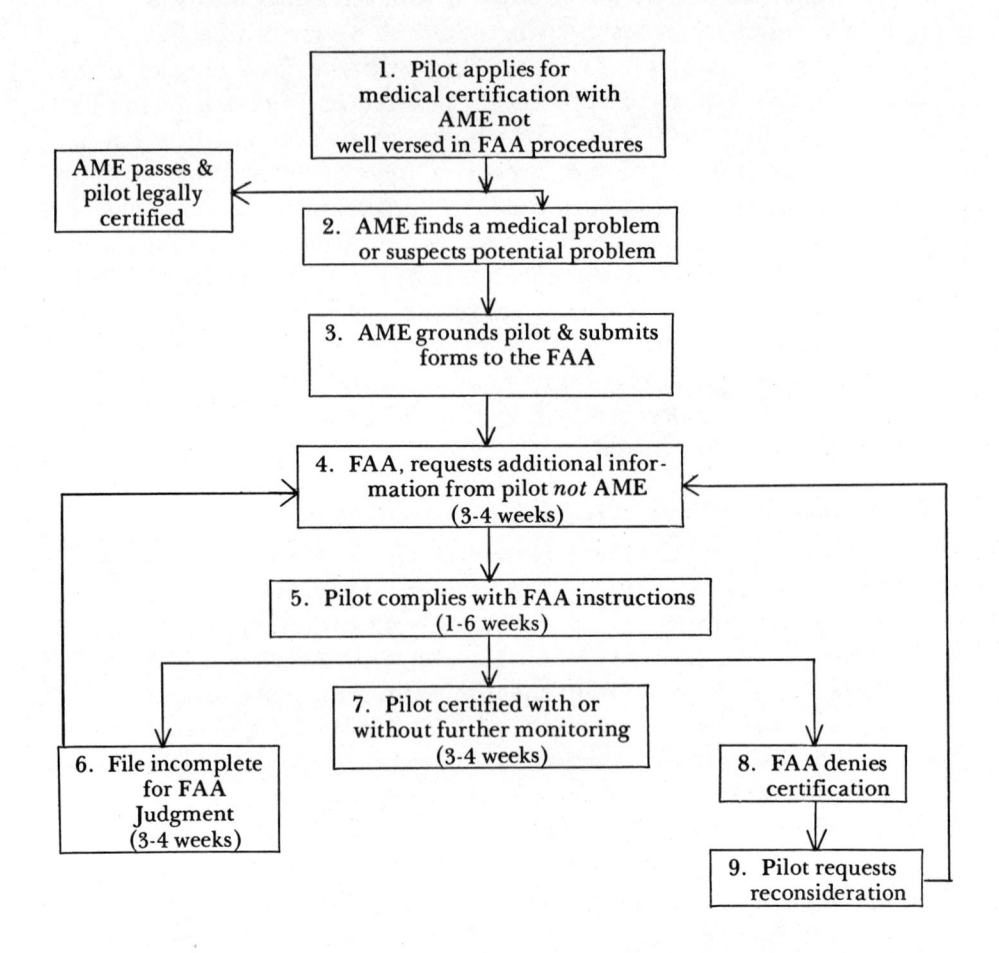

```
                    ┌─────────────────────────────┐
                    │ 1. Pilot applies for        │
                    │   medical certification with│
                    │   AME not                   │
                    │   well versed in FAA        │
                    │   procedures                │
                    └─────────────────────────────┘
┌──────────────┐                │
│ AME passes & │◄───            ▼
│ pilot legally│    ┌─────────────────────────────┐
│ certified    │    │ 2. AME finds a medical      │
└──────────────┘    │    problem or suspects      │
                    │    potential problem        │
                    └─────────────────────────────┘
                                │
                                ▼
                    ┌─────────────────────────────┐
                    │ 3. AME grounds pilot &      │
                    │    submits forms to the FAA │
                    └─────────────────────────────┘
                                │
                                ▼
     ┌────────►   ┌─────────────────────────────┐   ◄────┐
     │            │ 4. FAA requests additional   │        │
     │            │    information from pilot    │        │
     │            │    *not* AME  (3-4 weeks)    │        │
     │            └─────────────────────────────┘        │
     │                          │                         │
     │                          ▼                         │
     │            ┌─────────────────────────────┐        │
     │            │ 5. Pilot complies with FAA   │        │
     │            │    instructions (1-6 weeks)  │        │
     │            └─────────────────────────────┘        │
     │                          │                         │
     │             ┌────────────┼──────────────┐         │
     │             ▼            ▼              ▼         │
  ┌─────────┐ ┌──────────────────┐  ┌────────────────┐   │
  │6. File  │ │7. Pilot certified│  │8. FAA denies   │   │
  │incomplete│ │with or without  │  │certification   │   │
  │for FAA  │ │further monitoring│  └────────────────┘   │
  │Judgment │ │(3-4 weeks)       │         │             │
  │(3-4 wks)│ └──────────────────┘         ▼             │
  └─────────┘                       ┌────────────────┐   │
                                    │9. Pilot requests│──┘
                                    │ reconsideration │
                                    └────────────────┘
```

COMMENTS:
#1. The typical AME is not highly knowledgable regarding expeditious handling of problem certifications.
#2. Often AME does not tell pilot significance of findings - allows FAA to be "bad guy" & inform pilot he is grounded.
#3. Often prematurely submits report to FAA.
#4. FAA requires additional medical information to reconsider a pilot's fitness.
#5. Pilot sometimes left on his own to work with specialists & handle additional paperwork required by FAA.
#6. Because of misunderstanding concerning intent of further evaluation & requirements, FAA requests further data, pilot is back at box 4.
#8, 9. By this point pilot often finds himself trying to coordinate & achieve cooperation from 3 entities - the original AME, any specialists who have entered the picture, & the FAA.

Key to improperly handled sequence is not knowing & properly *anticipating* the FAA needs *in advance* of their requests. Tremendous amounts of time can be lost waiting for the FAA to respond to previous paperwork submission - only to learn more paperwork is necessary.

The FAA's Certification Process

PROPERLY MANAGED CERTIFICATION SEQUENCE

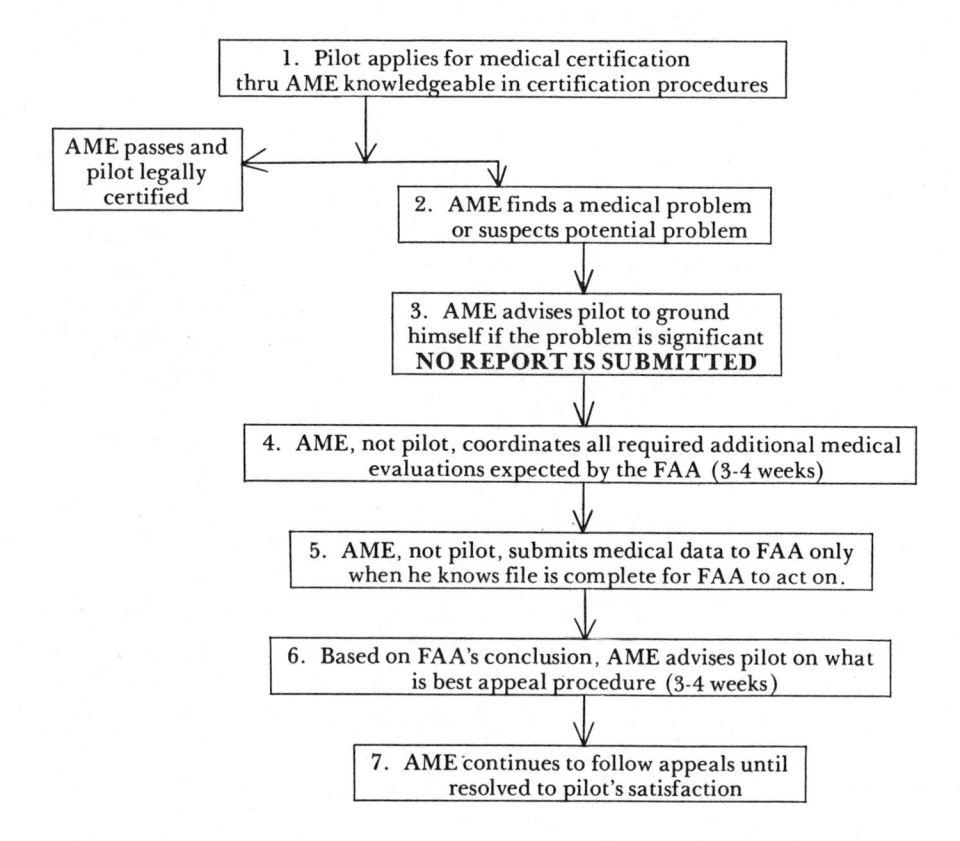

```
        ┌──────────────────────────────────────────────────────┐
        │  1. Pilot applies for medical certification          │
        │  thru AME knowledgeable in certification procedures  │
        └──────────────────────────────────────────────────────┘
                              │
┌──────────────┐              ▼
│ AME passes and│◄──┌──────────────────────────────────────┐
│ pilot legally │   │  2. AME finds a medical problem      │
│ certified    │   │  or suspects potential problem       │
└──────────────┘   └──────────────────────────────────────┘
                              │
                              ▼
        ┌──────────────────────────────────────────────────┐
        │  3. AME advises pilot to ground                  │
        │  himself if the problem is significant           │
        │  NO REPORT IS SUBMITTED                          │
        └──────────────────────────────────────────────────┘
                              │
                              ▼
        ┌──────────────────────────────────────────────────────┐
        │  4. AME, not pilot, coordinates all required additional medical │
        │  evaluations expected by the FAA (3-4 weeks)         │
        └──────────────────────────────────────────────────────┘
                              │
                              ▼
        ┌──────────────────────────────────────────────────────┐
        │  5. AME, not pilot, submits medical data to FAA only │
        │  when he knows file is complete for FAA to act on.   │
        └──────────────────────────────────────────────────────┘
                              │
                              ▼
        ┌──────────────────────────────────────────────────────┐
        │  6. Based on FAA's conclusion, AME advises pilot on what │
        │  is best appeal procedure (3-4 weeks)                │
        └──────────────────────────────────────────────────────┘
                              │
                              ▼
        ┌──────────────────────────────────────────────────┐
        │  7. AME continues to follow appeals until        │
        │  resolved to pilot's satisfaction                │
        └──────────────────────────────────────────────────┘
```

COMMENTS:
#1: This is the key to success of control: that the AME is knowledgeable in the certification process and aviation medicine, and is experienced in working with the FAA in protecting the healthy pilot's medical certificate.
#2: AME will try to anticipate potential problems which ban be resolved without compromising your responsibilities as a pilot.
#3: This is the second key to success: no report is made to the FAA until both the AME and pilot are satisfied with the file. If pilot's condition is not significant, pilot continues to fly.
#4: AME can make appointments with other specialists and already knows what the FAA will require for further evaluation. There is no need to wait for FAA's direction.
#5: AME submits entire file to FAA, with cover letter, rather than making the FAA the coordinator of the varied medical reports. AME may also alert FAA about coming file.
#6: AME can then determine what courses of action to follow once everyone knows what is necessary to satisfy FAA requirements.
#7: The AME should commit himself to the pilot to assist him thru the entire appeals process and explain why such actions are necessary.

Pilot's Manual of Medical Certification

plished, and, of course, the pilot gets caught in the middle again. There is no solution to this other than knowing your AME's philosophy of certification beforehand. The key question to be asked of any examining AME involved in your certification is "What does the AME do if he finds something wrong?" His response is an indication of his knowledge of you, your career, and the FAA, plus his willingness to work with you on your behalf.

Instead of ignoring the problem, the AME may give you some indication of your situation by saying, "I don't think you have a disqualifying problem and in my opinion the FAA should certify you, but the book says that I can't certify you because of 'x' result. I'll have to send everything in to the FAA and let them decide. Sorry." The AME will not issue the certificate at that time, but in any case, he drops the ball in the lap of the FAA and *you* must wait until the FAA gets around to passing judgment or requesting more data. You're in the middle again.

The situation I have just described, that is, letting the FAA resolve any problem, is the more common approach used by some AMEs. We have already discussed the consequences for you: Valuable time is lost unnecessarily, as is money invested in you by your company. Everyone gets defensive, but the only one hurting for a job is you, the grounded pilot. Once the 8500-8 is sent from the AME's office to the FAA, time is out of your control and the wheels of the bureaucracy begin their sluggish turning. The "passing the buck" philosophy may be common, but there is a better way. You obviously aren't qualified to play doctor, but if you know the system and how it *can* work, you will have better control of your future and will even be able to assist your AME should you develop a problem in your medical certification.

A SUGGESTED BETTER OUTCOME OF THE EXAMINATION

Let's go back to that place in the certification process where the AME has finished his evaluation and is ready to lay his judgment on you. Again, if all is OK *and for real,* that's the end of the process until the next exam is due. If, however, some abnormality is found, whether proven or suspected, the following sequence of events *could* take the place of "passing the buck." In other words, many of these "not normals" could be resolved quickly by competent hands. The following are ways by which the AME and the FAA can keep you flying, even with less than perfect results from a physical exam.

Limitations:

The AME finds a condition that is not perfect but he has the authority to issue you a certificate provided you adhere to certain *limitations*. The most common example is poor distant vision, which requires glasses or contact lenses to correct to perfect vision. The limitation, which is written on the front of your medical certificate, would then read, "Holder shall wear (or 'possess' in the case of poor near vision) correcting lenses while exercising the privileges of his airman's certificate." Limitations for other conditions may be placed on the certificate after further evaluation by authorities, not necesarily medical (such as check pilots), to demonstrate your ability to fly with the defect. Then, after being reviewed by the FAA, you are allowed to fly. The limitation becomes a *part of your certificate* and you must be able to prove you are following these limitations when flying. These limitations are "operational" limitations. There are also "functional" limitations whereby the FAA can limit the functions of the pilot to certain crew positions, i.e. "duties not to include pilot in command", "Valid for flight engineer only", etc. The FAA used to be able to limit a First Class Medical certificate but the courts have said that the FAA does not have this authority. The new amendment will allow for such functional limitations for second and third class medicals.

Waivers (or Statements of Demonstrated Ability).

If your medical condition falls in the range of suggesting a denial but is not necessarily detrimental to safe flying, the FAA (*not the AME*) may grant a *waiver*. You must prove that the presence of the problem does not interfere with safe flying. A waiver is most commonly used in cases of *very poor uncorrected distant vision* (worse than 20/100 for First Class), hearing not in the acceptable limits as stated in the guide, color vision deficiency, etc. A waiver differs from a limitation in that the medical criteria can be "waived" or foregone if it can be proven that the medical condition does not interfere with safe flying with or without correction. This is done by actually demonstrating your flying abilities to other examiners, again, not necessarily doctors. (A limitation, on the other hand, is what the pilot must do to be properly "equipped" to fly and meet regulations, such as wearing glasses. With a *limitation,* the deficiency must be corrected by some method while flying. With a *waiver,* the pilot's ability and experience compensate for the deficiency.) A waiver allows a pilot to fly by proving through his flying *ability* that his condition is not risky, even though he technically doesn't meet the letter of the AME's guide. A waiver is not a black mark on your record. It is actually protection granted by the FAA against being unnecessarily grounded by an AME regarding a specific condition.

A waiver is *not* what is given if you have a condition that is *medically* disqualifying and that *could* interfere with safe flying in the form of an unexpected and sudden incapacitation or distraction. Some examples of this include blood pressure that is too high, risks of having a

Pilot's Manual of Medical Certification

Medical Certificate and Statement of Demonstrated Ability

UNITED STATES OF AMERICA
DEPARTMENT OF TRANSPORTATION
FEDERAL AVIATION ADMINISTRATION

MEDICAL CERTIFICATE ___SECOND___ CLASS

THIS CERTIFIES THAT *(Full name and address)*
John Q. Public
800 Independence Avenue, S.W.
Washington, D.C. 20590

DATE OF BIRTH	HEIGHT	WEIGHT	HAIR	EYES	SEX
6-5-22	5'11"	165	Brown	Blue	M.

has met the medical standards prescribed in Part 67, Federal Aviation Regulations for this class of Medical Certificate.

LIMITATIONS: Must wear back brace while flying.

DATE OF EXAMINATION: May 3, 1970
EXAMINER'S SERIAL NO: 0001-08-8
SIGNATURE: *PV Siegel MD*
TYPED NAME: P. V. Siegel, M.D.
AIRMAN'S SIGNATURE:

FAA FORM 8500-9 (1-67)   SUPERSEDES FAA FORM 1004-1

UNITED STATES OF AMERICA
DEPARTMENT OF TRANSPORTATION
FEDERAL AVIATION ADMINISTRATION

STATEMENT OF DEMONSTRATED ABILITY
This form cannot be used in lieu of a medical certificate; it should be attached to your medical certificate.

AIRMAN'S NAME AND ADDRESS
John Q. Public
800 Independence Ave., S.W.
Washington, D.C. 20590

CLASS OF MEDICAL CERTIFICATE AUTHORIZED	WAIVER SERIAL NO.
SECOND CLASS	3 8 W 5 7 0 2 5

LIMITATIONS: Must wear back brace while flying.

PHYSICAL DEFECTS: Lumbosacral strain

BASIS OF ISSUANCE:
[ ] OPERATIONAL EXPERIENCE   [ ] SPECIAL PRACTICAL TEST   [X] SPECIAL FLIGHT TEST
[X] Special Medical Examination

FOR THE FEDERAL AIR SURGEON
DATE: May 3, 1970
SIGNATURE (TO BE SIGNED IN INK): *PV Siegel MD*
NAME AND TITLE (TO BE TYPED):
P. V. SIEGEL, M.D.
FEDERAL AIR SURGEON

FAA FORM 8500-15 (12-69) FORMERLY FAA FORM 779

UNITED STATES OF AMERICA
DEPARTMENT OF TRANSPORTATION
FEDERAL AVIATION ADMINISTRATION

MEDICAL CERTIFICATE ___THIRD___ CLASS

THIS CERTIFIES THAT *(Full name and address)*

SPECIMEN COPY

DATE OF BIRTH	HEIGHT	WEIGHT	HAIR	EYES	SEX
7-7-42	6'1"	175	Br.	Br.	M.

has met the medical standards prescribed in Part 67, Federal Aviation Regulations for this class of Medical Certificate.

LIMITATIONS: Holder shall wear contact lens (left eye) and shall possess correcting glasses for near vision while exercising the privileges of his airman certificate.

DATE OF EXAMINATION: May 3, 1970
EXAMINER'S SERIAL NO: 0001-08-8
SIGNATURE: *PV Siegel MD*
TYPED NAME: P. V. Siegel, M.D.
AIRMAN'S SIGNATURE:

FAA FORM 8500-9 (1-67)   SUPERSEDES FAA FORM 1004-1

UNITED STATES OF AMERICA
DEPARTMENT OF TRANSPORTATION
FEDERAL AVIATION ADMINISTRATION

STATEMENT OF DEMONSTRATED ABILITY
This form cannot be used in lieu of a medical certificate; it should be attached to your medical certificate.

AIRMAN'S NAME AND ADDRESS

SPECIMEN COPY

CLASS OF MEDICAL CERTIFICATE AUTHORIZED	WAIVER SERIAL NO.
THIRD CLASS	4 8 G 5 7 0 3 5

LIMITATIONS: Holder shall wear contact lens (left eye) and shall possess correcting glasses for near vision while exercising the privileges of his airman certificate.

PHYSICAL DEFECTS: Distant visual acuity:
(R: 20/20) L: Aphakic, corr 20/20 w/contact lens

BASIS OF ISSUANCE:
[X] OPERATIONAL EXPERIENCE   [ ] SPECIAL PRACTICAL TEST   [ ] SPECIAL FLIGHT TEST
[X] Special Medical Evaluation

FOR THE FEDERAL AIR SURGEON
DATE: May 3, 1970
SIGNATURE (TO BE SIGNED IN INK): *PV Siegel MD*
NAME AND TITLE (TO BE TYPED):
P.V. SIEGEL, M.D.
FEDERAL AIR SURGEON

FAA FORM 8500-15 (12-69) FORMERLY FAA FORM 779

heart attack or stroke, etc. For this category of conditions, the FAA passes judgment based on the additional *medical* data provided by you and your doctors which we will describe later in the chapter. You are certified to fly if the added *medical* data proves you are healthy enough not to sacrifice safety. Each case is evaluated and judged individually and on its own merits and risk factors. By realizing the distinction of these alternatives in resolving medical problems, you can assist your AME to act on your behalf and urge him to at least coordinate some of the additional evaluation that the FAA will require.

Until now we have been discussing less serious medical conditions, conditions that could be resolved through additional testing with the AME's assistance in working with the docs in Oklahoma City and advising the pilot on what action is necessary. Yet we are all aware of unnecessarily long delays for simple situations such as poor vision that was correctible to 20/20, when a waiver should be easily and quickly obtainable if handled properly. Although getting this supplemental data is your responsibility, your AME should know what needs to be done and he should be able to expedite the action for you. After all, that's what you are paying him to do and that's what the FAA expects from him when he is designated to be your AME. If your AME doesn't know what to do, either you or your AME can simply call Oklahoma City or the Regional Flight Surgeon in your area to get instructions on what to do without having to wait to be told by the FAA when it finally gets to your application. No names need be mentioned. There can be complete confidentiality while you are getting guidance on the next step. Just keep in mind FAR 61.53. Don't fly if you are not well and you and your AME won't have to report anything to the FAA until everything is in order.

Conditions that are Disqualifying

These are conditions that your AME has no authority to judge and must turn over to the FAA for consideration. There are nine conditions, discussed in Chapter 3, that are "mandatory" denials, by your AME that is, the regulations make no exceptions and even the Federal Air Surgeon has no choice but to deny you initially. The appeal process for these cases will be discussed later. But what we will discuss now is how the other disqualifying conditions—those other less serious, but numerous conditions listed in the AME's guide—can be certified. Although less serious than the "mandatory" denials, these are the conditions that cause the most problems in getting certified, create the most misunderstanding, and result in the greatest waste of time if not properly handled. If properly handled, these conditions should be resolved for you in a matter of a few weeks.

At this point, I want to discuss a little known part of the medical regulations, namely paragraph 67.19 of Part 67 "Special Issue: —". This is particularly important since the amendments of May 1982 now more clearly defines the authority of the Federal Air Surgeon. Prior to this amendment, the Federal Air Surgeon could issue a certificate (by FAR 67.19) to a pilot who did not meet the medical criteria, providing certain conditions were met which precluded any threat to safety—all conditions except the nine mandatory conditions described earlier. In other words, even the Federal Air Surgeon could not certify a pilot with one of these disorders, even if it could be shown that the pilot was safe to fly. This is where the "exemption process" came into being. That is, since the Federal Air Surgeon couldn't certify this safe pilot, a grant of exemption from the regulations was issued—an exemption not of the medical standards but from the restrictions of paragraph 67.19d. After getting around this restriction thru an exemption, the pilot's medical status was considered. This took 6-12 months or more, mainly due to the administrative requirements inherent in the exemption process.

With the new amendments, the Federal Air Surgeon no longer is restricted from certifying the "9 mandatory disorders" (See Appendix I). The revised Part 67.19 is self explanatory and only time will tell if the intent of these amendments are in the best interests of the pilot and flying safety. In any case, you will still need to provide the same medical information as described throughout the book. In other words, your responsibility to prove your fitness to fly hasn't changed. The intent now is for the Federal Air Surgeon to have the authority to certify you for *any* disorders—if you are fit to fly.

Before I get into details, let me once again state what I believe are acceptable methods of certification if everyone respects the other's responsibilities and obligations. **If you feel that there is any doubt that your medical condition is going to interfere with safe flying—don't fly. Ground yourself. The FAA doesn't need to know about your health until you are ready to go back flying. It's not illegal to be sick and not fly!** FAR 61.53 applies **only** if you fly. Your inherent concern is not the possibility that you will not always be healthy, it's what happens to you and your career when you and your "illness" are reported to the FAA. Your doctor should be able to tell you what you have wrong, why it is incompatible with safe flying, and what needs to be done to make you medically safe and acceptable to everyone. The FAA wants only medically safe pilots at the controls. Even if the FAA does not certify you right away, you will be many steps ahead of the poor pilot who is an innocent victim of the "pass the buck" process. In my judgment, there is no need to immediately report your condition to the FAA until you have everything in order—providing you defer flying until approved by the FAA. Again, this assumes you and your doc/AME are in control of your medical status, as you would be if under the military flight surgeon system. The FAA must be allowed to review the accumulated medical data *before* returning you to flying status. By getting *all* the required data to the FAA before your certificate application gets tangled up in the red tape of the bureaucracy, *you* have better control of getting back to flying.

There will be those who will ask, "what about the sick pilot who continues to fly?" Well, I am not talking about the turkey who doesn't trust anyone and wants to play doctor *and* FAA and then judge himself to be healthy. He is a menace to our colleagues and the public and I worry more about his sense of responsibility, logic, and attitude than his medical condition. There is enough redundancy in professional flying that his peers will be able to cover for him if he does become seriously ill while flying. Obviously, this pilot should be reported to someone, maybe to his peers first, but certainly to someone who can keep him from endangering himself and others. He is also ruining the credibility of those professionals who want to help and assist a *responsible* pilot in returning to flying status after he is well. Thankfully, this irresponsible pilot is in the minority, but he is still a part of our system. I feel that we must respect the *responsible* pilot who does not want to fly if he is ill (providing he actually is ill). His return to flying status should be handled by a doctor who knows how to help. That should be your AME!

There are also those who would criticize this approach by saying that the FAA requires that it be informed right away to keep the irresponsible pilot from flying. This is a valid consideration. That is why the FAA encourages (not demands) the AME to report sick pilots. The FAA knows that the majority of professional civilian pilots lack adequate medical monitoring and supervision, thus necessitating immediate disclosure. Therefore, as we discussed earlier, the lack of support of some of the AMEs has led the FAA to be more "possessive" of its responsibility to enforce the regulations and to protect the public from the minority of pilots who would abuse the privilege and responsibility of flying. Still, if you are not flying while you are being further evaluated and you remain self-grounded until the FAA acts on the medical data, no one is really breaking any rules. More important is the fact that the *pilot* remains in control of *his* future, instead of placing it entirely in the hands of the FAA. If your AME is unable or unwilling to "pick up the ball," then you have to rely on the FAA to tell you what to do. As mentioned before, it is *your* responsibility to seek the added data for certification, not the responsibility of the AME or the FAA. But you don't have to do it alone or wait for the FAA to respond. Tell the AME to hold your file until either he or you call the FAA for guidance.

If you and your AME feel that you are healthy enough to fly while the additional evaluation is going on, have your AME call the FAA for guidance. Initially, no names need to be mentioned and the FAA may simply approve your request if there is no compromise to safety. If they say no, simply don't fly. The FAA still does not need to know who you are, and you can go on to the next step.

On the back of the 8500-8 form, item #62, is the space for the AME to tell the FAA what course of action the AME is recommending after his exam. In most cases of *potential* denials, the "deferred" box is (or should be) checked, signifying that, although you may have a disqualifying condition according to the book, there could be added data to prove that you are not a menace in the skies. An AME will check this box but not add any data when he elects to "pass the buck" to the FAA. By doing this, he instructs the *FAA* to tell you what the next step is, such as to get additional data. The AME should know this next step and should provide the data *along with* the 8500-8 he submits. Checking the "denied" box could complicate the ease of re-certification.

There are cases in which it is obvious to the AME that the applicant shouldn't fly or in which the applicant himself knows he is grounded or even wants to be grounded. Then a letter of denial is sent to the applicant with a copy to the FAA. The FAA will review the data submitted by the AME and if indicated will confirm the denial with a similar letter. This official denial is important to the professional pilot to prove his "medical retirement" and to justify his claim to his insurance carriers. Instructions still are given to this grounded pilot for further appeal.

RE-CERTIFICATION FOR DENIED CONDITIONS

More medical data will be required for the FAA to make a decision about possible recertification of a disqualifying medical condition. With adequate documentation of additional tests and data that prove that the "abnormal" condition is *not* significant and would *not* jeopardize the safety of flying, most pilots eventually can be certified. Additional information is obtained from additional tests and examinations as instructed through supplementary evaluations. Remember, although these are instructions for the doctors you will be seeing, you are the one to whom these instructions are sent. The FAA can't tell you what doctor to see, but your AME can suggest whom he thinks could help.

These protocols instruct the doctors who will be doing these evaluations, who are not necessarily AMEs, on what the FAA requires— *strictly* requires.

One would think that these specifications are straight-forward, but failure to follow these instructions is one of the areas where the recerti-

The FAA's Certification Process

DEPARTMENT OF TRANSPORTATION
FEDERAL AVIATION ADMINISTRATION

SPECIFICATIONS FOR NEUROLOGIC EVALUATION

I. If not previously submitted, all records are required covering prior hospitalizations and/or other periods of observation and treatment. These records must be in sufficient detail to permit a clear evaluation of the nature and extent of any previous neurologic disorder. Medical release forms are enclosed for you to complete and send to the physicians and/or hospitals which hold your records. You should request that copies of your records be mailed directly to this office. Please date and sign one of the release forms and return it to us for our records. An envelope is provided for this purpose.

II. A report by a qualified neurologist is required. (A "qualified" neurologist is preferably one who has been certified by the American Board of Psychiatry and Neurology or by the American Board of Neurological Surgery, or one who has the background equivalent for Board certification. The applicant's personal physician is often a good source for such a referral.)

The neurologist's report must supply the following:

1. Detailed report of a recent neurological examination.

2. Pertinent X-rays, electroencephalogram with activating procedures*, cerebrospinal fluid examination, or other tests and laboratory procedures as may be indicated.

A petitioner with a history of neurologic disorder who seeks exemption from Part 67 of the Federal Aviation Regulations on the basis of full recovery must submit the reports and objective evidence as listed above. In instances of cerebrovascular disorders the petitioner must be free from all symptoms for at least two years before his petition will be considered by the Panel.

*These procedures are utilized to elicit a latent abnormality in brain rhythm and are of special value where the resting record has shown no change from the normal. The standard techniques are hyperventilation, sleep and photic drive. Generally three minutes of hyperventilation and a period of recording during drowsiness and sleep are included in a standard tracing. The sleep may be spontaneous or induced by chloral hydrate or barbiturates. Drugs used in the activation procedure, including dosages, should be indicated in the report.

AC Form 8500-11-1 (6-69) Supersedes previous edition   FAA AC 70-5038

Pilot's Manual of Medical Certification

DEPARTMENT OF TRANSPORTATION
FEDERAL AVIATION ADMINISTRATION

SPECIFICATIONS FOR PSYCHIATRIC AND PSYCHOLOGICAL EVALUATION

I. If not previously submitted, all records are required covering prior psychiatric hospitalizations and/or other periods of observation or treatment. These records must be in sufficient detail to permit a clear evaluation of the nature and extent of any previous mental disorders.

II. A report by a qualified psychiatrist. (A qualified psychiatrist is preferably one who has been certified by the American Board of Psychiatry and Neurology, or one who has the background equivalent for Board certification). The applicant's personal physician is often a good source for such a referral.

The examination must be of recent date and the report should be in sufficient detail and depth to permit an accurate evaluation of the petitioner's interval history and his current psychiatric status. Conclusory statements alone are not acceptable. All pertinent medical records and professional reports should be made available to the psychiatrist prior to the preparation of the report.

III. A report by a qualified clinical psychologist who is experienced in administering such tests. (A qualified psychologist is preferably one with a state license or certification with a Ph.D. in Clinical Psychology, or is listed in the National Register of Health Service Providers in Psychology). The applicant may contact the local psychological association for a referral.

The report (including a copy of the test protocols) should contain a detailed psychological evaluation based on a battery of psychological tests. Such a battery should include: (1) the Rorschach, (2) the complete Wechsler Adult Intelligence Scale (WAIS), and as considered appropriate by the practitioner, any two of the remaining tests or their equivalents:

    a. Bender-Gestalt
    b. Draw-A-Person
    c. Thematic Apperception Test (TAT)
    d. Minnesota Multiphasic Personality Inventory (MMPI)
    e. A Sentence Completion Test

FAA Form 8500-26 (10-78)

The FAA's Certification Process

DEPARTMENT OF TRANSPORTATION
FEDERAL AVIATION ADMINISTRATION

CARDIOVASCULAR EVALUATION SPECIFICATIONS

These specifications have been developed by the Federal Aviation Administration (FAA) to determine an applicant's eligibility for airman medical certification. Standardization of examination methods and reporting is essential to provide sufficient basis for making this determination and the prompt processing of applications. This cardiovascular evaluation, therefore, must be reported in sufficient detail to permit a clear and objective evaluation of the cardiovascular disorder(s) with emphasis on the degree of functional recovery and prognosis. It must be performed by a specialist in internal medicine or cardiology and should be forwarded to the FAA immediately upon completion. Inadequate evaluation or reporting, or failure to promptly submit the report to the FAA, may delay the certification decision. As a minimum, the evaluation must include the following:

I. **MEDICAL HISTORY.** Particular reference should be given to cardiovascular abnormalities —cerebral, visceral, and/or peripheral. A statement must be included as to whether medications are currently or have been recently used, and if so, the type, purpose, dosage, duration of use and other pertinent details must be given. A specific history of any anticoagulant drug therapy is required. In addition, any history of hypertension must be fully developed and if thiazide diuretics are being taken, values for serum potassium should be reported. A comment should be included on any important or unusual dietary programs.

II. **FAMILY, PERSONAL, AND SOCIAL HISTORY.** A statement of the ages and health status of parents and siblings is necessary; if deceased, age at death and cause should be included. Also, an indication of whether any near blood relative has had "heart attacks," hypertension, diabetes or known disorders of lipid metabolism must be provided. Smoking, drinking and recreational habits of the applicant are pertinent as well as whether a program of physical fitness is being maintained. Comments on the level of physical activities, functional limitations, occupational and avocational pursuits are essential.

III. **RECORDS OF PREVIOUS MEDICAL CARE.** If not previously furnished to the FAA, a copy of pertinent hospital records as well as out-patient treatment records, with clinical data, x-ray and laboratory observations and copies of or original serial EKG tracings, should be provided. Detailed reports of surgical procedures as well as cerebral and coronary arteriography and other major diagnostic studies are of prime importance.

IV. **GENERAL PHYSICAL EXAMINATION.** A brief description of any comment-worthy personal characteristics; height, weight, representative blood pressure readings in both arms; funduscopic examination of retinal arteries; condition of peripheral arteries; carotid artery auscultation; heart size; rate; rhythm and description of murmurs (location, intensity, timing, and opinion as to significance) and other findings of consequence must be provided.

V. **LABORATORY DATA.** As a minimum, must include actual test values of:

A. Routine urinalysis and complete blood count.

B. Blood chemistries (values and normal ranges of the laboratory).

FAA Form 8500-19 (3-77) Supersedes Previous Edition

(OVER)

1. Serum cholesterol and triglycerides after 12- to 16-hour fast.

2. Blood uric acid after 12- to 16-hour fast.

3. Fasting blood sugar. If the fasting blood sugar is elevated, include at least a three-hour glucose tolerance test following glucose loading for the three preceding days.

4. Blood urea nitrogen.

5. Protein-bound iodine, if indicated, and reports of any other diagnostic studies which may have been recently performed.

C. Recent PA and lateral chest x-rays (provide films if abnormal).

D. Electrocardiograms.

1. Resting tracing.

2. Exercise stress test.

a. State methodology used.

b. Provide blood pressure determinations at rest, at each stage of the exercise stress test, and during the recovery period.

c. Submit representative EKG tracings for the control, exercise and recovery periods.

d. Obtain recovery EKG tracings until there is a return to the control configuration and/or until the control level of heart rate has been achieved.

NOTE: The information obtained through a determination of current cardiovascular capacity and an evaluation of strain end points under the stress of rhythmic exercise is considered essential to the determination of fitness of any applicant with suspected or known cardiovascular disease. Current practice indicates that a stress test on a treadmill, using either Bruce or Balke protocol, is optimum in providing the desired performance data. Alternatively, an ergometer test that results in a degree of work of approximately 85 percent of the age-predicted maximum capacity using heart rate end points is acceptable. All usual medical precautions should be followed in prescreening, election to test, testing, and follow-up on applicants who undergo exercise stress testing. The resting tracing should be reviewed by the examining physician for evidence of acute coronary insufficiency, recent myocardial infarction, or repolarization abnormalities. EKG evidence of recent, unsuspected myocardial change or infarction would contraindicate exercise testing. Please state reasons if the exercise stress test is medically contraindicated.

☆U.S. G.P.O. 1977-725-165/514

fication process gets held up, and *you* get caught in the middle. Some doctors do not agree with the FAA's instructions for evaluating a medical disorder and would rather fight the system than provide the required data. That is one of the bureaucratic charms of the FAA. Some of your doctors may be correct in thinking the way they do, but whether or not a specified test is commonly used by the medical community in which you will be getting your evaluation is not important. What is important is that the FAA requires it. Usually, if something is not performed according to the protocol, the FAA will not consider the appeal favorably. Trying to "fight city hall" for the sake of winning a scientific medical opinion is yet another place where *your* career is compromised. It seems much more realistic to me for my colleagues to swallow scientific pride, provide the FAA with what it wants, and get the job done swiftly. If your doctor feels that even more *additional* data would be in your best interest, great. But don't ignore the minimums set by the FAA, and tell your doctor not to ignore them.

Remember, the usual response by the FAA to an *incomplete* workup and file is, "Based on the information provided, we cannot certify your condition." It gets denied but perhaps it could have been certified if *all* the data were initially provided. It doesn't make sense to take short cuts in the certification process when a career is at stake.

Another question that you and your AME must consider in choosing doctors to do your evaluations is, which are medically reputable and best qualified to provide data that will be accepted and respected by the FAA? This is truly a problem and the individual pilot must rely on knowledgeable AMEs for advice. After all, most pilots do *not* frequent or need other doctors and specialists. The Airline Pilot's Association provides an aeromedical "coordinator" within its local union structure and an aeromedical physician at the national level of the union who specializes in directing grounded pilots to appropriate consultants. (The union does not pick up the tab for the consultant's fee.) This is a valuable service to airline pilots who have no other resources. Air carriers with medical departments also can provide the services necessary to keep their pilots flying.

So the time has come when the AME says, I can't pass you because of "X" condition. At this point, the AME may tell you why "X" is disqualifying (unsafe for flying) until proven otherwise, plus what needs to be done to satisfy the requirements of the FAA. Unfortunately, to adequately explain such a career-threatening situation to a pilot, who is understandably scared, takes a lot of time; time that most doctors don't have. This is another reason the AME might defer the decision concerning your certificate by sending the 8500-8 to the FAA and waiting for its reaction. For now, let's assume that the AME is willing

Pilot's Manual of Medical Certification

to act in your behalf and begins the process of obtaining the necessary additional data. The AME should be aware of what the FAA requires and "open the door" to consultants who appreciate what needs to be done. Ever try to get an appointment with a specialist as a new patient? It takes weeks or months!

Let's use an example to clarify the order of events so far. Your AME finds that your blood pressure is consistently too high. He explains the situation to you, areomedically and legally, and he elects to treat you with a blood pressure medicine acceptable to the FAA. He knows that it is harder to get you certified if he puts you on medication. So he coordinates the needed specialists and labs for the reports and tests listed in the Cardiovascular Protocol. Much time can be saved if the AME collects all the data, puts it into a neat file, and *then* submits this to the FAA. Forcing the FAA to be the coordinator greatly prolongs the process. Once this data is obtained, it is sent to Oklahoma City for the FAA's review and judgment. The FAA must pass judgment on the information supplied by your AME. If the file is complete, the FAA can make a decision as soon as it gets to an FAA doctor. However, as stated earlier, there may be many weeks between the arrival of your application and evaluation by an FAA doctor. If the file has enough data to justify that the medical condition would not jeopardize the safety of flying, the FAA doctor will certify you. In doing this, he must consider the data, whether or not your condition is a risk, and how you intend to use your medical certificate. If the doctor does not feel that you are safe to fly, he will send you a letter of denial, but he will also include in the letter instructions on the next step toward certification should you want to take it.

The reason for the alternatives, including the right to further appeal procedures, is either that the Oklahoma City doctor does not have the authority to pass judgment even though the data is adequate, or that the Oklahoma City doctor doesn't feel that you have a certifiable condition. You may still have a strong potential for being certified, but you must take your application to the next step, that is, *you must request* reconsideration by the Federal Air Surgeon in Washington. This does not happen automatically. The information can be reviewed by the Federal Air Surgeon, who has the authority to either decide in your favor, ask for more data, or deny you. Yet, even with his denial, the Federal Air Surgeon will suggest a course to follow. The key point is that the Federal Air Surgeon must accept the responsibility of determining whether or not your medical condition is safe for flying. If the problem is more complex than the Federal Air Surgeon wants to safely judge, he will call upon a board of specialists for further interpretation. In other words, the decision is not an arbitrary one and every attempt is made to be fair, while considering the top priority in the mind of the Federal Air Surgeon: the effect of your medical condition on

The FAA's Certification Process

safe flying. Remember, the practice of medicine and how your health affects your ability to do any job is like weather forecasting, not an exact science, and the data are subject to interpretation. Critics of the system may have a valid point but are not responsible for insuring safe flight.

If the Federal Air Surgeon's office decides against certification because you do not meet the requirements of the FARs (such as the nine mandatory denials) then the next step used to be to request an *exemption* to the FARs. That is, you were stating that, although strictly speaking you did not meet FAA's standards, you and your doctors felt that there was no problem present or that the problem was not a danger to flying. Your request to be exempted from the FARs was a request, in effect, that the FAA write a new regulation especially for you.

Now, with new amendments to the medical FARs in effect, the exemption process is no longer necessary. However, the *medical* criteria remain the same. Since the Federal Air Surgeon now has the authority to deny or certify even the nine mandatory denials, a thorough evaluation and documentation is essential. It is here that many detailed reports are absolutely necessary for your medical file. Several competent opinions are helpful. Although the FAA will make its *own* conclusion based on the data presented, your doctor's opinion is also considered, especially if he is known and respected by the FAA. Often, however, your family doctor, acting in *your* best interests, may state that he sees no reason for you not to fly when, in fact, he is not thoroughly knowledgeable of how your medical condition affects your flying performance. This could mislead you into thinking your problem is less of a danger than it actually is. Therefore, the doctor you choose should be knowledgeable about aviation medicine and the certification process to express a respected opinion regarding your condition and flying. Pilots in a union can get important information and assistance from their aeromedical advisor, a specialist in aviation medicine, knowledgeable in FAA certification and respected by FAA doctors. Those without a union's help must seek out for themselves the necessary assistance from competent aeromedical consultants.

All the data are organized into your file in Washington for presentation to the board of specialists. It makes it easier for the FAA if all the material is complete and organized when it is sent in, and if it is easier for the FAA that is one more step in your favor. These data are then discussed by the board of doctors, all specialists in their fields (such as cardiology, internal medicine, neurology, etc.). They are also knowledgeable about the effects of these medical conditions on the safety of flying and the chances of there being a problem in the future. Remember, you are considered a risk to flying if you have a medical problem that is serious, and the burden is on *you* to prove to the FAA's doctors that your condition will not interfere with safe flying.

There can be several conclusions by the board of doctors:
1. More data are needed, perhaps because they weren't included or weren't requested. Thus no decision would be made.
2. You would be certified with some type of monitoring of your medical condition and possibly a time limit of validity.
3. You would be denied because the data were not adequate to justify certification; had there been a more complete presentation of data, you might have been certified.
4. You would be denied, either because all the data possible to obtain are present but you are not considered safe for flying, or because the risk of developing a worse problem is great.

It should be obvious that before you present your case to the FAA you should have obtained as much medical data as are necessary to reach a realistic conclusion. Don't second-guess the FAA! Even if your request for reconsideration or exemption is denied, you can go to the NTSB (National Transportation Safety Board). However, this is an expensive, prolonged ordeal since it now becomes a legal issue of interpretation. In other words, since medicine is not an absolute science and there can be several viable and professionally acceptable opinions, the NTSB allows for the two sides (i.e.: your side and that of the FAA) to "battle it out" in a hearing. Both sides are represented by their attorney. Before taking this action, be sure you have obtained competent medical *and legal* advice regarding your ability to fly safely with your condition. What you are doing, through an attorney, is claiming that the FAA is wrong in its decision to deny you and that you have exhausted all possible interpretations for review of the FAA. For example, say you had a mild stroke. All the current tests, x-rays, angiograms, and other sophisticated data indicate a "clean bill of health." The FAA will base its decision on its statistical evidence that those who have had a history of stroke have a greater chance of having another. Since your case could be equivocal in determining potential risks for future flying, the FAA will deny you, to be on the safe side. If, on the other hand, you have gathered a commendable collection of data, along with superb legal counsel with expert witnesses, you can challenge this denial to the NTSB (or higher). (The NTSB can't *change* the standards) Even if you win your medical back be advised that the FAA can appeal the decision and also has the option to keep a close eye on your file. Also be aware of the 60 day period after a denial during which you must *file* (not necessarily carry out) your appeal. A formal denial is required *before* you can file. A competent attorney well versed in aviation medicine and law could be a real asset if all else fails. In my opinion, however, this legal route should be used only as a last resort. There are few cases which truly need to be appealed to the NTSB — if you have actually sought certification properly as described earlier.

The 1982 amendments allows for more flexibility for second and third class medical certification. Both classes can now have functional limitations which allows a pilot with a medical disorder to fly, who would otherwise not be certifiable. This means that by restricting the medical to specific crew positions, this pilot can fly although not truly medically qualified for unrestricted flying. This limitation does not include first class medical certification. In addition, third class medical criteria will be much more lenient as noted in Part 67.19c (see page 137).

I am not implying that if you follow these suggestions, you won't have any problems with the FAA. That would be naive and too good to be true. However, the more *you* can do to better your case and improve your appeal, the greater chance you will have of a positive result. Certainly you will be way ahead of your colleague with the same medical problem who is waiting for someone else to act.

In conclusion, the process of certification may be delayed by two main problems:

1. The inherent bureaucratic sluggishness in review, evaluation and judgment, and in the administrative process of informing you. You have no control over this bureaucratic delay and you must wait it out like everyone else.

2. Failure on the part of yourself and your doctor to submit all of the necessary, complete data as required by the FAA in an optimal amount of time. This you *can* control by following my suggestions.

Therefore, in those areas where you can have control, *take* control. And try not to get too frustrated by those areas that are out of your hands. Better still, avoid this situation in the first place by practicing a good health-maintenance program. Here again, there are some important and critical areas of your health over which you have control — and some that you don't. Let's take control of those areas in which you have something to say. That means getting back to health maintenance, knowing what your medical status *truly* is, and developing a prevention philosophy.

4

Specific Health Problems and Flying

A 38-year-old airline pilot admits that he is more than usually apprehensive about his FAA exam. He likes snacking, laying around, watching TV and drinking beer. When his doctor "suggested" he watch his habits because his blood pressure was "creeping up" a bit, the combination of all of this was too much. He busted his next FAA exam because of high blood pressure. Many months later, in better shape and watching his diet, his blood pressure was controlled, but only with medication. He is flying, but every year he has to prove to the FAA that his hypertension is under control.

THE FOLLOWING TOPICS are the most common medical factors that affect a pilot's health and his medical certificate. Alcoholism is also a major factor and will be discussed in chap. 9. You should become knowledgeable about this material since no pilot is immune from any of these problems. These include:
Blood pressure and hypertension
Diabetes
Coronary artery disease
Vision
Hearing
Cardiovascular evaluation and heart stress testing

Blood Pressure and Hypertension

Elevated blood pressure is one of the more frequent "common" medical conditions that can ground pilots for weeks or even years. The continual pumping of blood through the blood vessels exerts a certain amount of pressure against the inside walls of the arteries and veins, pushing outwards just like the hydraulic system in your aircraft. When the pressure becomes too high, it can damage the arteries, the organs supplied by them, and the pump itself, the heart. This **persistent** increase in pressure is known as hypertension.

Specific Health Problems and Flying

Blood pressure is determined by listening to the sounds of flowing blood in an artery of the arm with a stethoscope using a tight cuff around the upper arm and a gauge called a "sphygmomanometer." Using this method, your doctor can measure your blood pressure *at that time*. It is not necessarily your *true* "every day" pressure. Many factors influence your blood pressure readings: emotions, fears, environment, position, posture, temperature, time of day, the sight of the medical office, the comments by the doctor, to name a few. So, a *diagnosis* of hypertension should never be based on only a few readings. Instead, many should be taken over a period of time involving several visits to find out whether the pressure really is up *all* the time and not just at one particular moment. Sometimes the mere act of repeating blood pressure readings or an idle comment such as, "how long has your blood pressure been up?" can keep a professional pilot's blood pressure elevated whenever he is in the doctor's office, though it may return to normal as soon as he leaves. Your blood pressure during a simulator check ride from "checkitis" is probably the same with "examitis" — high!

If your AME takes one blood pressure reading or even several, and they all are elevated, this may not necessarily be the "hypertension" that the FAA is concerned about. High blood pressure from *stress* is much different than high blood pressure from disease (hypertension). The FAA, in fact, wants your *recumbent* blood pressure — taken while you are lying down — which gives you the benefit of determining your best blood pressure. Also, the FAA will accept a higher blood pressure than your own doctor will accept. Blood pressure in excess of 140/90 is often treated by most doctors with medication, whereas the FAA will *accept* an *un*treated blood pressure of 140/90 for a 35-year-old pilot.

Simply establishing the fact that a certain pilot has "hypertension" or high blood pressure is not the sole concern and does not define the whole problem. Having the high blood pressure may be a manifestation of a disorder that is *causing* an elevation in pressure. It is that process that must be corrected or reversed. The *cause* may be a dietary abuse which can be altered easily, or it may be more serious such as a stricture (sudden narrowing) of an artery, or a kidney dysfunction. In any case, it needs to be corrected before any more damage is done by the increased blood pressure. Hypertension is dangerous, even though you may not have any symptoms. The working environment in which you fly — dry air, sedentary activity, dehydrated, hypoxic, being "geared-up" for an emergency — can seriously aggravate even mild hypertension. That elevated "hydraulic pressure" is bound to blow out sometime.

There is a misconception that a person with hypertension is "hyper" or "tense." That is not the medical meaning of the word.

Pilot's Manual of Medical Certification

FAR 67.31 (e) (4)

(1) Class I:

Age Group	Maximum readings (reclining blood pressure in mm)		Adjusted maximum Readings (reclining blood pressure in mm)[1]	
	Systolic	Diastolic	Systolic	Diastolic
20-29	140	88	—	—
30-39	145	92	155	98
40-49	155	96	165	100
50 and over	160	98	170	100

[1] For an applicant at least 30 years of age whose reclining blood pressure is more than the maximum reading of his age group and whose cardiac and kidney conditions, after complete cardiovascular examination, are found to be normal.

(2) Classes II and III: Blood pressure above 170 mm. of mercury systolic* or 100 mm. of mercury diastolic.

*"Systolic" blood pressure is the highest "hydraulic" pressure within your blood vessels. "Diastolic" means the lowest, or resting, pressure before going back up to the systolic level.

Also, hypertension is not limited to fat people. The skinny, calm fellow may also have the same hydraulic pressure problem going on inside his circulatory system and need the same treatment.

It is common knowledge in the aviation world that many professional pilots consult their own family doctors for illness and then their AMEs *only* to get by their flight physicals. This defeats the real purpose of the flight physical (are you safe to fly?); it's like cramming for an aviation exam and then forgetting and disregarding the vitally important information when it is over. This practice, although understandable, can be especially threatening to your career because of the usual way that hypertension is treated in most medical communities. If your own doctor is not familiar with the FAA's criteria, you could be in for a long ordeal in regaining a medical certificate that is denied because of a single elevated blood pressure in your AME's office or your own doctor's office. For example, let's say that your family doctor (not your AME) sees you and says that your blood pressure is "up a bit," or you had a friend take it, or had it taken in a drugstore, or at some sports club. The point is, if your blood pressure is up, it needs to be checked out and treated. Keep in mind that many pilots will see their own doctor for treatment and then see their AME for certification. Your own doctor may do a few tests to check you out more thoroughly. That's good. I hope he will measure your blood pressures over several days before tagging you with a *diagnosis* of hypertension. As I said earlier, in many pilots' cases the mere mention of an elevated blood pressure will be enough to cause an otherwise normal blood pressure to go up as soon as the pilot sees a blood-pressure apparatus or a white coat. I hope your private doctor will take this into account before becoming too aggressive in his evaluation and therapy. Nevertheless, your doctor can't ignore the fact that your blood pressure is elevated, regardless of the conditions under which it was taken. Recent medical evidence indicates that even mild hypertension (140/90) should be treated. An aggressive doctor could put you on medication for a blood pressure that is acceptable to the FAA. So what's the best treatment for a *pilot?* Your doctor can't ignore your high blood pressure because he knows it is dangerous to your health. Your family doctor—*if* he knows you're a pilot—is in a true dilemma. How to treat your hypertension without grounding you? The most important answer is that treatment should not be limited to medication.

It is common knowledge that among an inherently *healthy* population, such as pilots, there is a direct relationship between increased blood pressure and smoking, increased weight, too much salt, lack of exercise, alcohol, caffeine, etc. It is also realized by the medical profession that the odds of the usual patient successfully giving up cigarettes, decreasing alcohol consumption, eliminating unnecessary foods that he likes, cutting down on coffee, and beginning a good exercise program are between zero and none. And the typical doctor has little time to try to explain why it is important to avoid these abuses. But the increased blood pressure is still there, so the doctor says, "take this medicine once a day and see me in a couple of weeks," knowing the odds are better that the patient will take the pill—which is the easy way out—than that he will change his habits. He may casually add, in passing, "Try to lose some weight and watch the cigaretts," but there often is little time spent in explaining how or why.

The blood pressure may be controlled by the medication, but then you have two strikes against you. First, you have a diagnosis of hypertension, and second, you are using medication to control it. *Both are disqualifying* until further evaluated and judged by the FAA. In other words, the FAA rightfully assumes that you have tried all other measures of controlling your blood pressure, such as losing weight, avoiding salt, cutting out cigarettes and so forth, but to no avail, and that medications are the *only* way your blood pressure (hypertension) can be controlled. The FAA also reasons that this *could* mean that you have *severe* hypertension (because of your *need* for medication) and therefore they want to determine what else could be wrong, such as with the heart, kidneys, brain, etc. So, the FAA will ask for the "FAA's cardiovascular evaluation," which is very comprehensive and could open the door to more unexplained, yet abnormal data—data that now *must* be reported to the FAA. A good physical *is* important, but why *have* to report it?

The irony is this: Your increased blood pressure may not be serious at all and could be controlled simply by avoiding those abuses you *should* be avoiding anyway, whether you're hypertensive or not. This is another reason for trying to stay ahead of the game by maintaining the good health you brought to the profession.

Having a career that does not allow you to have hypertension or take medication would seem adequate reason for you to follow some commen-sense measures of maintaining a good physical condition and protecting that valuable career. Yet a pilot's inherent apathy probably will cause him to continue being out of shape until an elevated blood pressure cannot be ignored any longer. Therefore, should your doctor tell you that your blood pressure is up and he wants to try some medication, ask him if you could *try* some other measures first, since medication could jeopardize your career. These measures include:

1. No smoking. I say again. NO Smoking.
2. Reduce your salt (salt is *sodium* chloride) intake. *Sodium* is the culprit in this case—it's also found in preservatives and in other parts of food, not only in ordinary table salt.
3. Maintain an ideal weight, a weight your family doctor or your AME should be able to define.
4. Avoid caffeine, which is a *very* strong stimulant to the heart and makes it work harder than it has to.
5. Avoid alcohol in more than moderate amounts. The *stimulant* effects to the heart of excessive alcohol can last for days.
6. Develop an exercise program that is appropriate for *you,* but under the supervision of a doctor.

As you can see, there is nothing magic about these measures and nothing that you shouldn't *already* be doing. By following this very basic program, you greatly reduce the chance of developing an elevated blood pressure as well as many other health problems that would not be acceptable to the FAA, your AME, or your family doctor. I can't say this enough: Waiting for your doctor to tell you that you have something wrong, in this case your elevated blood pressure, is not the best way to pay attention to maintaining your health. The odds are great that if you abuse those social amenities in which our society overindulges, some disorder will catch up with you. Granted, there is a percentage of pilots who are overweight, smoke and drink too much, and somehow still come through their exams. But the odds for this are small. "Playing the odds" in Los Vegas provides an immediate response. "Playing the odds" with your health will not show results for years. If you want to play those odds, that's up to you; but they're against you! Common-sense measures like watching your diet, can improve the odds, and your blood pressure usually can be controlled. Better still, you can keep it from being elevated no matter what the stressful circumstances. By the way, *I* can abuse my health, take medication and go back to work. You can't!

Don't assume you can take your health for granted by waiting for hypertension to develop, and *then* work out some way to keep your medical certification. I have worked with too many pilots whose hypertension *eventually* was controlled easily (by common sense measures), but the pilot spent many months, and even years, getting back on the line.

Diabetes

Diabetes is the inability of your body to metabolize or efficiently use *essential* sugars as fuel. Sugar (to the body) is sugar—no matter what the *source* is. Ultimately, *all* "sugars" (to the body) is metabolized as *glucose* which *is* common sugar. As a result of this inability the entire body is subject to potentially serious complications.

This disorder probably is one of the best-recognized diseases but one of those least understood by the medical profession. It would appear that the more doctors investigate this disease, the less they know about it. There is no doubt that diabetes represents a *multitude of different* problems occurring at the same time within the body, all of which are *deteriorating* processes unless brought under control. Therefore, the presence of diabetes severe enough to require medication (that is, *not* controlled by diet) *is* a real risk to safe flying.

As far as the FAA is concerned, diabetes is initially ruled out by doing a urinalysis "dipstick" test during your AME's certification exam. This simply tests your urine for the presence of sugar by a color change on a strip of chemically treated paper. This is, at best, a screening test and the absence of sugar by that test does *not* totally rule out the presence of diabetes nor diagnose a *potential* diabetic pilot. But, by the same token, if sugar is present in the urine, then diabetes *must* be ruled out (for you and the FAA) by additional testing.

There is one disorder called renal glycosuria, which means that your kidneys "spill" or excrete sugar into the urine under *normal* circumstances. This is usually an acceptable medical variation once diabetes has been ruled out. The only way to determine this is to do additional special blood studies, which include a fasting *blood* sugar (the measurement of sugar in the *blood* after a minimum of eight hours without any food) and a glucose tolerance test (the hourly measurement of sugar in the blood and the urine following the ingestion of a specified amount of glucose). Both of these tests usually are adequate to define either the presence or absence of diabetes. However, there are situations where the results are equivocal, that is, the presence or absence of diabetes still cannot be determined absolutely, therefore the FAA may *require* a glucose tolerance test.

The glucose tolerance test is a controversial evaluation since it has a tendency to over-diagnose. For example, there are some people thought to have diabetes who in fact do not. The diagnosis for these people was based primarily on the glucose tolerance test results, which appeared to be abnormal but were not. In spite of the controversy, the FAA still requires a glucose tolerance test to rule out the presence of diabetes *if* it is suspected. Should you ever be asked to take a glucose tolerance test, be sure that you eat a "glucose tolerance test loading diet" during the three days prior to taking the test. Ask your doctor for the specifics. Keep this in mind: The results of the test are subject to interpretation by a physician *and* the same test results could have as many different interpretations as the number of physicians evaluating it.

As far as the FAA is concerned, there are upper limits for *blood* sugar; your own doctor may or may not consider those limits acceptable. A known diabetic *can be certified* if his diabetes can be controlled by diet alone; that is, with no use of oral medication or injectable insulin. The FAA quite reasonably assumes that if your diabetes is so severe that it *requires* medication, all other measures, such as diet control, have not worked. It also assumes that there will be other, inevitable complications.

Therefore, should there be *any* suspicion of diabetes by your own doctor or by your FAA examiner, it behooves you to make the utmost effort to follow a strict diabetic diet to give yourself every possible chance to control it *without* medication. Once your doctor decides that you must remain on medication, that could be the end of your flying career.

I have seen several cases where sugar has appeared for the first time in the urine of a pilot who has an extra amount of fat around him, overindulges in pastries and is generally out of shape. He feels good. Almost invariably, with better control of his dietary intake of carbohydrates, loss of weight and exercise, this tendency to "spill" sugar can be reduced and no further action is necessary. In other words, diabetes was *not* present, but the presence of sugar in the urine was a result of poor diet. Finding sugar in your urine and proving *to the FAA* —not just to you and your doctor—that you do not have diabetes is no way to get your attention if you know you are out of shape.

Coronary Artery Disease

Coronary artery disease (CAD) is one of the major causes of both permanent and temporary medical certificate denials. FAR's use the term coronary **heart** disease which to you means about the same. The current FAR Part 67 states that even a *history* of coronary artery disease requires *mandatory* certificate denial by your Aviation Medical Examiner. There is good reason for this, since anyone with coronary artery disease **does** have a greater risk of developing a heart attack or other disabling conditions leading to sudden incapacitation. Once coronary artery disease is detected through *any* means, it cannot be ignored-CAD is a **progressive** disease. These rules put the professional pilot in a quandary. If he has no symptoms relating to his heart, should he avoid looking for something that may ground him? Or should he look for something with the idea that if a problem does turn up, he will correct it to save his life and his health?

Coronary arteries are the vessels which bring necessary blood to the heart *muscle*. Heart muscle is like any other muscle in the body and requires oxygen and nutrients to function. The heart is simply a pump in the body's hydraulic system—and you only have *one* pump. This hydraulic system is a closed system in which arteries take oxygen and nutrient-rich blood to all parts of the body and blood is brought back to the heart via the veins. Coronary artery disease is either a plugging up of coronary arteries or a stiffening of the walls of the arteries, greatly compromising the ability of the arteries to bring blood to the heart muscle. If there is too little blood and therefore inadequate oxygen and nutrients, either chest pain (angina pectoris) develops or a myocardial infarction (heart attack) occurs.

Most medical professionals generally agree that coronary artery disease is a result of an abnormal amount of cholesterol either *within* the wall of the artery or causing formation of "plaques" or obstructions along the *inside* of the walls of the artery. Whether or not this cholesterol in the coronary arteries is directly related to the amount of cholesterol in your **blood** is a subject of much disagreement, but there *is* a direct relationship between the amount of cholesterol in your blood and the *risk* of developing coronary artery disease. Thus, knowing cholesterol levels, along with other test results, is a very important part of determining *your odds* of developing coronary artery disease in the future.

Many good books and articles refer to the relationship of cholesterol and other various factors in the development of coronary artery disease. My purpose is not to duplicate these efforts but to state basic facts, and let *you* come to your own conclusions and course of living.

Recognized risk factors, that is, those abuses that greatly increase the *odds* of developing coronary artery disease—and of a professional pilot losing his career—are: age, increased weight or obesity, increased blood pressure (or hypertension), cigarette smoking, family history of coronary artery disease, poor cardiovascular (heart) conditioning, high cholesterol, triglycerides, and other fats in the blood. Only two of these variables is beyond your control—the heritage of a family history of coronary artery disease and your age. Variables *you* can control are obvious to everyone even minimally versed in good health maintenance.

Consider this: If the *treatment* for a person with high blood pressure or coronary artery disease is weight control, the avoidance of cigarettes, alcohol, caffeine and high-fat foods, and the development of a good exercise program, why not begin such therapy *before* developing the disease that could take away your certificate? You would be doing nothing more than using common sense. This does require effort, but unfortunately you picked a career that requires you to maintain your health. I don't think you need the bureaucratic FAA to take away your certificate and force you into following a good common-sense health maintenance program to regain it when **you** could keep from losing it.

It *must* be realized that anyone with *known* severe coronary artery disease cannot safely fly an airplane. This is because, at altitude, oxygen partial pressure is reduced, adding even more stress to the heart muscle than already is present because of the CAD, and the potential for heart failure is increased. This is a controversial subject since there are prominent physicians who will say that there is no added risk. In any case, if you can control *risk* factors that are likely to lead to CAD and likely to end your career, it would seem prudent to begin to work on some sort of health-maintenance program now. It is very common to see a pilot develop hypertension or CAD solely as a result of allowing his physical condition to deteriorate. Some studies say that if we did angiograms on all our population, a significant percentage already would have CAD *without* symptoms. Many times this unsuspected CAD is found indirectly as a result of testing for an unrelated problem, such as high blood pressure. High blood pressure *requires* exercise cardiac stress testing for certification by the FAA, and the stress test is often the *first* indication that CAD is present. I am not advocating ignoring a medical problem, but if a doctor is forced to look for one, chances are he will find something wrong and if he has to report this to the FAA, your career is on the line. Therefore, if you can avoid hypertension by following a common sense health-maintenance program, *additional* tests (that could lead to discovery of other problems not medically significant) will not be necessary. I refer you to the last section of this chapter on cardiac stress testing to illustrate how many a pilot is grounded for *unsuspected* disorders when, had he just followed some common-sense health maintenance, he could have avoided the problem.

Bypass surgery, a medically common procedure for correcting (but not curing) CAD, is a subject important to professional pilots. It is very uncommon for a pilot with a history of a heart attack or significant CAD to regain a medical certificate allowing him to fly in *any* seat of responsibility, especially in the left seat of an airliner. Bypass surgery, which involves bypassing the clogged coronary artery with another implanted vessel (actually a leg vein), does, in fact, improve blood *flow* to that part of the heart muscle. However, it does not remove the initial *cause* of the progressive CAD. While the surgery will not cure CAD, it will improve one's status of health and "feeling good." Only time will tell whether or not this surgery removes the future risk of incapacitation. Therefore, the FAA will reconsider someone who has had bypass surgery; depending upon the results, passage of time, and whether or not he has been able to control other risk factors. Keep in mind, however, that this individual *still* has a history of significant CAD and still has the disease and therefore has a mandatory denial by his AME until further evaluation.

A key point bears repeating once again. CAD is a common problem in our society and it alone can ground you. Don't wait to be told you have CAD before you follow the common-sense treatment of watching for and controlling your risk factors.

Vision

Testing your visual acuity, that is, your ability to clearly see near or distant objects (with or without glasses), obviously is an important part of determining your ability to fly proficiently. All of you have had enough vision tests to know what the procedure is. However, there are occasions where the instrument (other than an eye *chart*) used for determining visual acuity could distort results because this instrument uses a series of mirrors to simulate distance. Therefore, if you have borderline results, make sure that your examiner has your vision checked either by using an eye chart in a well-lit eye lane or by referring you to an ophthalmologist or optometrist.

Most abnormal vision changes occur before age 20, and your vision might even improve during the next few years that follow. But after that, your vision will remain relatively stable, especially your distant vision. As you pass 40, your *near* vision will begin to deteriorate and "reading" glasses will be necessary. Your first indication that there may be a change is during night flying—the charts will be harder to read. Distant vision is pretty well fixed by age 25. The correction for abnormal near vision is meant for reading, to allow you to focus on a book or newspaper without too much difficulty. Keep in mind that as a pilot, much of your "near" vision work is at the instrument panel, the console or pedestal, and where you normally look at your approach plates. This location could be several feet further than the distance at which you hold books. Consequently, you should let your eye doctor know that you are a pilot so that he can prescribe two sets of glasses, one just for flying and one just for reading. Bifocals are also available where the correction is at the *top* of the lens for looking up at the overhead panel.

Glasses always have been accepted by the FAA as long as they adequately correct your visual deficiency. Deficient vision up *through* 20/100 is acceptable when corrected without any additional evaluation. For First Class certificates, vision poorer than 20/100 will require an eye evaluation by an eye doctor for a test called "refraction." This is a technique by which the eye doctor can determine the actual status of your eye to focus without correction. In most cases, the FAA will certify a pilot with a bad uncorrected vision as long as his corrected vision is 20/20 and the "refraction" is within acceptable limits.

Contact lenses worn by a pilot while flying required a waiver until a few years ago. They now are considered to be in the same class as frame glasses and do not require a waiver.

Glaucoma and testing for glaucoma are highly misunderstood, because tonometry is not specifically required for airline pilots. The tonometry test uses a delicate instrument that gently touches the eye to determine the pressure **within** the eyeball. (The drops used to "deaden" the feeling of the cornea do *not* dilate your eyes and will not interfere with driving or flying.) As pressure increases in the eye of a patient with glaucoma, it will gradually destroy his retina and his ability to see. This is a *permanent* change leading to progressive blindness. If you wait until *you* begin to notice changes in your vision rather than be tested for glaucoma, the damage may have already begun. However, with this simple, routine tonometry test, an early pressure increase can easily be detected and treated *before* it is too late.

Glaucoma that has been brought under control with eyedrops before the vision has deteriorated is certifiable by the FAA. Many pilots are not only reluctant to have this eye test, but will also refuse to go to a doctor that does it because they feel that it is unnecessary and fear that if they do have early glaucoma, their careers are finished. Actual-

Specific Health Problems and Flying

ly, their careers would be jeopardized *only* if they have advanced glaucoma that was not detected in time for treatment. These misinformed pilots rationalize that it is better not to know that they have glaucoma at all until it is so severe that they can't pass the visual-acuity test. This is a perfect example of ignoring a correctable problem until it becomes *uncorrectable*. Glaucoma is a disease that you should not put off treating until the very last minute, because at the very last minute it will be beyond correction and you will not be able to be certified.

"Color blindness" is not really an acceptable term any more. We now know that there are variations in color vision, and it is now referred to as "color deficiency." It is usually a permanent, unchanging condition. The main purpose of the test is to determine if you, as a pilot, are able to detect red and green, especially at night. Are the red and green lights in front of you approaching or departing? The runway approach lights are often red and green, VASI is red, etc. Therefore, the *screening* test usually used in a doctor's office is to determine the presence of color deficiency severe enough to compromise safety. If you miss a certain number of plates in the test, you are considered color deficient. There is also a more accurate test using different colored lights at different intensities, called "Color Threshold Test" which may show that you are color deficient—yet color safe. This test is usually done only in the military, unfortunately. For a Second or Third Class medical certificate, the FAA will allow a waiver if you can pass a "light gun test." This test simply determines whether or not you can distinguish between red and green by using a light gun, as used in an ATC tower. However, for a First Class medical certificate, a more critical evaluation is required. A flight test must be done. The examiner will fly with you in various conditions during the day and night, making sure that you can distinguish the VASI, radio towers, approaching traffic, etc. If you can, there is no problem with the certification. If you can't, then obviously you shouldn't be flying at night anyway. All these additional tests must be authorized by Oklahoma City *before* you take them. Your AME can assist in this coordination.

Depth perception testing once was considered to be an important part of your visual evaluation. Depth perception (having both of your eyes working together to determine the distance of objects) is only critical up to about 20 feet. Beyond that, depth perception is based on "visual cues." That is, over the years that you have lived, your eyes and your brain have become familiar with the *relative* sizes of different objects; for example, if you see a distant tree with a car next to it, you know the approximate size of each and are able to judge how far you are from them. This is why the 747 looks so slow while it is flying. Your brain's "computer" is not used to that large an aircraft and it appears to be closer and thus slower than it really is. However, if you flew a 727 at the same speed right underneath a 747, the relative increase in size of the 747 would be most apparent, and you would see more obviously the 747's *true* distance and speed. Along with this, different visual cues used to preceive an object on a clear day may be masked by haze, fog, etc. The main point is that depth perception testing is not as critical as one would expect, unless there is marked inability to "fuse" the eyes for vision less than 20 feet. This is what is called binocular vision, where both eyes are focusing on the same object, and is easily evaluated at the time of the physical exam and can be corrected by glasses.

"Space myopia" occurs while flying at altitude on a clear day. In other words, you have nothing distant to focus on, such as a cloud, when you look out the window. If you find yourself staring out the window, move your eyes around more and look around the cockpit occasionally, *plus* looking back at the wingtip. By not focusing on something distant, you may not be able to see a distant object clearly if it does appear, such as traffic not pointed out by ATC.

A lot is said about "Ortho K" (orthokeratology). This is a technique of using a special kind of contact lens that physically molds the cornea of the eye. The result in some is improved visual acuity when the contact lense is removed. Obviously, this is a popular technique for young pilots wanting to be hired by a company that accepts 20/20 only. Unfortunately, this correction is temporary, at best, and it *is* a "correction." So the burden is still on that pilot to state whether or not he has "uncorrected" 20/20. I guess it's worth a try.

Hearing

The ability to hear is as important as your vision. Although some of today's flying is done with black boxes, your sense of hearing still cannot be replaced for coordinating your flight with that of others in your airspace. And unlike your visual acuity which deteriorates with age and usually can be corrected with glasses so you still end up with 20/20 vision, the same is not true with hearing. Hearing aids are not compatible with safe flying nor can they correct poor hearing. Therefore, the *preservation* of your hearing is most important.

For the professional pilot's career, only the voice range is important: 500 to 2,000 cycles per second. Your airplane's communication system is not "high fidelity." That is, it is not burdened with the ability to communicate the higher and lower frequencies beyond the voice range. That is why the FAA only looks at the voice range in its evaluation. As long as you have acceptable hearing in the voice frequencies, you could be totally deaf in the others. That is, in fact, what often happens in high-frequency hearing loss.

The only true way to evaluate your hearing is with the audiogram. The "whispered voice test" is archaic and gives you no objective, quantitative data. The audiogram must be done properly in a quiet room with an adequate, well-calibrated instrument. The audiograms performed in most doctors' offices are screening tests at best, and if you suspect any hearing loss, it would be best if you had your hearing checked by an audiologist, someone who specializes in the determination of hearing ability.

Although the FAA is interested only in the voice range, you and your AME should also be interested in the higher frequencies. If a high-frequency hearing loss is detected, it is an indication that you probably are being subjected to excessive noise, because high-frequency hearing loss is most often the result of exposure to noise. This is an indication of a *progressive* process. In the past, flight surgeons often could determine the type of flying machine World War II aviators were flying, whether they were in fighters or bombers, and what crew position they flew, based on the degree of their high-frequency hearing loss and which ear was affected. In today's aviation, only those that must make the walk-around are really subjected to prolonged noise unless one flies his own airplane, uses chainsaws, lawn mowers, home woodworking equipment, etc. If your high frequencies are being lost through exposure to noise, this will progress and in time will pull down the rest of the frequencies, including the voice range. In time, with prolonged exposure to noise, the voice range looked at by the FAA will become unacceptable. The *only* way that you can detect this progression is through a well-performed audiogram.

Hearing loss from noise, which probably accounts for the greatest percentage of hearing loss in the pilot, can be prevented easily by the very simple and unsophisticated methods of using ear plugs and ear defenders. A change may be insidious and the only way you can be made aware of it is by an adequate audiogram.

How do you tell if you are in an area noisy enough to produce hearing loss? An area that will subject you to some hearing loss probably is best described as any area in which you must raise your voice above a normal speaking level for any length of time. Loss of hearing is prevented easily by wearing ear plugs or ear muffs, especially when exposed to extremely loud noise. Don't forget to use these even in your home activities. There is a product called "Ears," a sponge-rubber type of ear plug, which I have found to be most effective and comfortable. It is inexpensive and it is very easy to carry a pair in your flight bag. By the way, prolonged exposure to noise is very fatiguing.

When doing physical exams on pilots, I often ask them if they have ever had an ear block. There is either a very passive "no" or a very emphatic "yes!" This should show you what a "true believer" is, for those who have ever had an ear block never want another one. Ear blocks occur quite commonly when flying with a cold. There is nothing "macho" about being able to fly in the presence of the common cold. An ear block occurs because of the inability of the eustachian tube to equalize pressure on both sides of the eardrum. As the aircraft and cabin altitude-climb, the pressure decreases within the middle ear. With an earblock, air going out of the middle ear quite easily escapes through the congested eustachian tube. However, on descent, the air cannot get back through the congested eustachian tube and a negative pressure results within the middle ear. The external increase in pressure on the outside of the eardrum now begins to push it inward, creating severe pain plus an additional ear block as a result of the swelling created by the block itself. If you are caught in this situation, you should relieve the block immediately, if it is at all possible, by returning to an altitude above that at which the earblock began. That is, bring the cabin altitude back up beyond where you were level and then slowly decrease the cabin altitude. The valsalva maneuver will assist—hold your nose and then blow against that resistance. There are other techniques that people use, such as cracking their jaws, swallowing, shaking their heads, etc. The important point is that the pressure must be equalized before reaching ground. Otherwise, severe damage can result. If someone feels he can take a chance and fly with a cold, then develops an ear block once on the ground, he can develop a block that may require weeks to resolve. The pilot is definitely temporarily grounded if he has an ear block. Some of the oral decongestants that can be bought over the counter, such as "Sudafed," are quite effective if you know that you have a mild congestion. Be sure the "decongestant" has *no antihistamines* because antihistamines can cause drowsiness. Read the label. Some of the nasal sprays, especially those long-lasting ones, can be kept in your flight bag if you feel you have an ear block developing. These should only be used sparingly since overuse of nasal spray can create its own congestion because of irritation.

A sinus block is similar to an ear block except that the sinuses are involved. The sinuses are located over the forehead and on both sides of the nose around the cheek bone. Again, anyone who has had a sinus block does not want a repeat performance. The same techniques are used with sinus blocks as for ear blocks.

There is a considerable amount of personal awareness of ear wax. Some feel that it is absolutely mandatory that all traces of ear wax be removed and will use all sorts of techniques to get it out, everything from toothpicks and hairpins to flushing with water. However, grandma's old rule of "Use nothing smaller than your elbow to stick in your ear" is still important. Unless the wax is obstructing the entire lumen of the ear canal, the wax actually is there for a purpose. It prevents foreign bodies, such as dust, bugs, etc. from entering, and it provides its own ear plug for reduction of trauma by noise. If you are a scuba diver, however, the wax can form a dam and water can be held behind it. As with flying, and for the same reasons, one should never dive with an ear block or with a cold and doubly so it you have ear wax present. The rule that you should never dive a certain number of hours before or after a flight is for the same reason: changes in external environmental pressure.

The FAA's Cardiovascular Evaluation and Cardiac Stress Testing

If your AME and/or the FAA determine during your routine FAA exam that you may have a cardiovascular problem (i.e. elevated blood pressure, abnormal EKG, etc.), the FAA will require additional medical data before it will certify you. This more thorough physical is outlined in the FAA's protocol for a "cardiovascular evaluation." It is not routinely done unless there is a suspected problem.

This FAA cardiovascular evaluation is like any other *comprehensive* medical evaluation by your own doctor. Such complete physicals usually include a thorough history and a physical examination. In addition, a chest x-ray and battery of blood tests and resting EKG are common. *This kind of evaluation is essential in any good health-maintenance program.* But this evaluation must be sent to the FAA because *they* requested it. Based upon these data, the doctor usually is able to make a fairly valid interpretation of your over-all health. With that as a basis, your doctor might add more-elaborate tests to evaluate any suspected medical disorders more completely. However, an additional test in the *FAA*'s cardiovascular evaluation is required—the cardiac-exercise stress test. The stress test, although a very valuable medical tool, is subject to considerable controversy depending upon with whom you are talking and within what medical community you have the test. At this point I would like to make it perfectly clear that the opinions expressed now are my own. In addition, I am in no way advocating that a potential or suspected cardiovascular disorder be ignored. However, each time a physician evaluates a patient, he considers the effectiveness, the necessity, the risk factors and the economics involved, along with the element of time, before subjecting the patient to these sophisticated tests solely to determine a diagnosis. It is common knowledge that there are many medical tests available that can tell us a lot, but some are extremely expensive and complex and therefore are not done routinely. Some of these tests add a risk factor and are reserved for special medical problems. Using this philosophy to determine the necessity of any test for an individual, you must consider that in a professional pilot's situation a cardiac stress test is potentially threatening. Part of a doctor's Hippocratic oath is that he will do no harm. A stress test might ruin a pilot's career. Therefore, consideration of a stress test must weigh its effect on a pilot's career against its need in the diagnostic process. The reasoning for this is simple. AN ABNORMAL—(OR POSITIVE)—STRESS TEST IS AN INDICATION OF A HEART DISORDER UNTIL PROVEN OTHERWISE. Yet, it is a medically accepted fact that up to 20 percent or more of cardiac stress tests that are considered abnormal are actually found to be free of any abnormality *after* subsequent and more sophisticated tests are done. Most people—those who don't fly for a living—return to work **during** these subsequent tests. A pilot, however, can be grounded until the suspected disorder is ruled out.

Keeping this in mind, let us discuss the cardiac stress test and its implication on a pilot's career. Stress tests basically are performed for three reasons: when your doctor suspects that you have a diseased heart or a potential problem with your cardiovascular system; before beginning an exercise program, and for screening purposes in a preventive medicine. It is important that the technique of a stress test be the same for whoever performs it so that all results have a comparable meaning. Basically you are connected by a series of wires to an EKG machine so you can be monitored at all times with a continuous tracing during exercise. The doctor then makes you work. That is, he increases the resistance on the bicycle or raises the incline of the treadmill so you *must work* harder, which consequently increases your pulse rate. The Masters Two Step stress test is inaccurate for these purposes. The doctor, before the test, will have determined a "target rate" based mainly upon your age. As you work harder, the heart's pumping rate goes higher. As this is happening, the doctor is watching the monitored EKG and looking for abnormalities such as a change in the regularity of the heart beat, blood pressure and your symptoms. He is not simply looking for how long or fast you run. At the same time, he is looking for depression of the ST segment. (a portion of the EKG tracing which indicates how the heart is functioning **electrically**) The ST segment should not become depressed by your being put through this exercise even up to the target rate. Once you have reached this projected target rate without ST segment depression, the stress test can be diagnosed as being basically normal. (The stress test should be done in facilities capable of taking care of cardiovascular emergencies. People with unsuspected heart problems have had cardiac arrests or equally serious problems during the test. Therefore, facilities must be available for resuscitation.) If no ST depression is noted, everything is OK, assuming no irregular rhythm develops. However, if the ST segment does depress, what does that mean? As mentioned, it is considered abnormal until proven otherwise, depending upon why you were there, what sort of symptoms you have, and the status of your complete physical condition. The doctor may elect to do additional tests. The doctor may repeat the test, get a second opinion, and after still equivocal findings, may still subject you to more elaborate sophisticated and expensive tests such as a Thalium scan and the ultimate test, the coronary angiogram.

Of course, the perfect evaluation would be obtained by opening you up and looking at the coronary arteries as during an autopsy. These arteries are the source of blood which brings oxygen to the heart muscle. We are concerned about any one or all of these arteries in this cardiovascular evaluation. All the tests—except physically looking at the arteries and the coronary angiogram—are implicit tests. That means we "imply" the condition of the coronary arteries by the tests we have done. Stress tests are simple screening tests in most cases and are not as effective in determining the condition of the arteries as the Thalium scan and the angiogram. Currently, the angiogram is the *only* test that can determine the true status of your coronary arteries and that's what you have to prove to the FAA—that your coronary arteries are not significantly diseased. However, in all vocations but one, an individual can go back to work even though he is being further evaluated. The exception, of course, is you, the pilot. If you have an abnormal stress test, you may be grounded until it's proven that the results are not disqualifying for flying duties—and it often is difficult to determine just how much a doctor must subject you to in order to rule out coronary artery disease.

Knowing this, why would a pilot undergo a stress test? Well, first of all, most pilots are interested in their health, and therefore some will occasionally get into an exercise program like those at the YMCA's, athletic clubs or schools. People running conditioning programs suggest that you have a stress test before beginning, to determine the physical condition of your heart and to protect you and them from an unsuspected heart problem. Usually this means that your own doctor should certify that there is no indication you couldn't follow the conditioning program. The stress test usually is an appropriate way for him to make such a recommendation.

Another reason for the stress test is the pre-employment or company physical exam. Again, this would detect unsuspected heart disease which could show up at a later date. A resting EKG would not rule out many such problems.

Yet another reason for the stress test is the FAA cardiovascular evaluation. As you know, a resting EKG is required by the FAA at age 35, and then annually after age 40 for a First Class certificate. If you have an abnormal EKG or a change in your resting EKG, the FAA will want the cardiovascular evaluation. Another reason would be if you have hypertension (high blood pressure) or other suspected heart problems.

So far there is no big deal about taking a cardiac stress test, but there is that klinker—the false positives. Therefore, all this evaluation (for a false positive result that could not be ignored) could come about because of high blood pressure or other *controllable* problems that would likely result from your poor physical condition.

As I mentioned before, I am not advocating ignoring a medical disorder. However, most responsible pilots are not ignoring their health, and as a part of their job must have periodic examinations. They are way ahead of the general population in determining the status of their health. If we are following good health maintenance you and I don't need a stress test to confirm our heart or physical condition. If you can keep a step ahead of the situation, then the chance of your having an unsuspected heart problem is very small. If handled properly, there should be no threat in the stress test. However, if you have allowed yourself to be in a situation where a stress test is required and that stress test happens to be a false positive, there is only one person to blame for being grounded, especially if that test proves something you have always suspected—that you are out of shape.

So what do you do? A stress test is important. It can be a valid test, but it can have a direct bearing on your flying career. If it is required by the FAA, there is nothing that you can do. Just keep your fingers crossed and hope that everything works out. Be sure, however, that it is supervised by a knowledgeable AME who is familiar with the FAA's criteria and the interpretation of the stress test. But as I mentioned before, don't wait for this evaluation to be thrown at you as a result of your poor physical conditioning. If you intend to begin an exercise program, which I advocate, the necessity of a stress test should be determined by your doctor, who should know about the FAA criteria. He may feel that, all things considered, the stress test is not appropriate and not indicated to determine your status. However, in view of your physical and medical condition and your age and the type of program you are starting, the doctor may require the stress test. If this is the case, then I would certainly agree with this necessity, especially if the doctor suspects a cardiovascular disease.

The most important thing of all is to learn and to remember what could develop from a test that need not have been done. So let me repeat the key points of the stress test: It is a valid tool and definitely has its place, but it is a subjective interpretation and can have false positives. By keeping ahead of yourself, you can avoid an unnecessary stress test *that must be reported to the FAA*. Be sure that your doctor is informed about the criteria you must meet and the impact that a false positive will have on your career. An abnormal stress test cannot be ignored since it is an indication of cardiac disorder until proven otherwise, and it could be a cause for unnecessary grounding.

Specific Health Problems and Flying

With the exception of the stress test, the cardiovascular evaluation is useful information for you. It is essential in evaluating your *true* health and to either confirm your good health or detect a potential progressive disorder that may, if untreated, lead to being grounded prematurely. It's an important evaluation, but wouldn't it be better to *not* have to report all this to the FAA?

5

How to Work With Your Family Doctor and Your AME

A 33-year-old pilot had some mild chest pain on his left side. His resting EKG was "slightly abnormal." His cardiac stress test was also "slightly abnormal." The doctor, who was terrified of flying, told the pilot that, although he didn't have a heart attack, he had a heart problem and would never fly again — in his judgment — although he was not an AME. The pilot, believing this, and being completely discouraged, grounded himself and did not seek guidance from an aeromedical doctor for several months. Once he did, however, further studies and interpretation by an aviation-oriented physician convinced the FAA that the pilot did not have a disqualifying or unsafe disorder.

WE COME NOW TO THE SECOND PART of the book. You now know why you must be healthy, how your health affects your flying performance and being a safe pilot, and how the FAA certifies your good health. Now you need to put that knowledge to work.

An obvious reason for a professional pilot's health-maintenance program is to increase his longevity so that he can keep flying until age 60. Staying alive and healthy until your 60th year plus one day may be a secondary challenge to you, but being able to remain productive at *any* age is more important. What benefit does a retired pilot receive from saying that he has made it to age 60 if he can't do anything productive with the rest of his life with this good health? The benefits of your health-maintenance program go beyond your goal of reaching 60. Whether flying for a living or not, continued good health is the key to a productive, rewarding, fulfilling life and keeping this in proper perspective, with realistic priorities, is a challenge. As a pilot, you are truly behind the proverbial "rock and a hard place." But there is a way out.

I stated earlier that it is relatively common, understandably, for a professional pilot to seek medical care or medical interpretation of his health from his family doctor and then seek FAA medical certification from another, non-threatening, FAA examiner: "If I feel OK, why look for trouble." The reason, of course, is the fear of losing your medical certificate and your career—no small matter. This could, however, cause a dilemma for the pilot who does have a medical problem even if unsuspected or without any symptoms. Your family doctor has a responsibility to you and so does the FAA examiner. However, as we have discussed earlier, your family doctor usually is not aware of your unique aeromedical requirements, the FAA requirements, and the affect of the medical disorder and its treatment on your safe flying performance. In contrast, your FAA medical examiner probably doesn't know much about you since you were reluctant to tell him anything more than you absolutely had to in order to pass your FAA physical. Let me use an example of hypertension (high blood pressure) to explain this "triple-standard dilemma"—**your standard** of health since you feel OK, your **doctor's standard** of health if he is looking for a problem, and the **FAA's standard** of health for you to fly. I use hypertension as an example since it is a very common occurrence and involves a medical disorder with which we are all familiar, one that often leads to a grounded pilot. The sequence of events is the same for any medical problem known or suspected.

If you have high blood pressure which has been determined through various sources available for taking your blood pressure (such as your family doctor, druggist, other physicals, etc.), your own doctor will probably treat you immediately with medication. Why? Because although most doctors realize that with a religious health-maintenance program such as weight loss, avoidance of salts, no cigarettes and so on, your blood pressure would likely be normal. Your doctor also knows from experience that most patients won't comply with this program, and he has little time for the futility of prescribing it. He can't ignore the hypertension, and he must treat you, so he puts you on medication. He does this because medication will lower your blood pressure, and you will take it more readily than you will follow a health-maintenance program. But this medication, along with the presence of high blood pressure, is disqualifying in the eyes of the FAA until more completely evaluated. A competent AME, however, may notice that the blood pressure is elevated, but will also notice that you probably are out of shape and overweight. He will suggest that these problems be corrected before the use of medication so that your blood pressure can be controlled enough to meet the FAA's requirements.

Since your AME is not commonly consulted if you have an illness, let's discuss how you can work with your own family doctor in preparation for your exam by the FAA no matter what the disorder is.

We will first discuss how a physician in private practice, that is, your family doctor, usually functions. His primary purpose and concern is to protect your health and treat anything that interferes with maintaining it. Secondarily, he is just as anxious to get you back to work as you are. Quite frequently, the doctor will treat his patient, and when he feels that the patient can work will tell the company that the employee can return to work with or without any restrictions. That note from the doctor is usually adequate justification to the company to allow him to return to work. The doctor has the credentials and the authority to do this. This is not true for pilots. Just because your doctor says you can return to work and there are no restrictions in *his* judgment, that does not mean that you have met the requirements of the FAA as I have previously defined. There is a great difference in having a medical disorder that is *treatable* to your doctor's satisfaction and a medical disorder that is *certifiable* to the FAA's satisfaction. That is, many disorders that are controlled may not necessarily be aeromedically safe for flying.

The practice of medicine is similar to meteorology. It is not an exact science, and varied interpretations of medical data is a limiting factor. The doctor will use his training and expertise and experience with other patients with similar symptoms to evaluate and treat you. You usually see your family doctor only when you have some symptoms that you cannot explain. His first objective is to review the symptoms for which you are seen (such as an ache, swelling, fever, etc.), and must first diagnose the *cause*. Then, based upon that diagnosis, he will treat you with appropriate medication or other therapy. Depending upon the severity of the illness that he suspects, the doctor may use as many tests as he feels necessary to evaluate the problem. If he still can't explain symptoms that could indicate a more serious disorder, he will do even more tests and probably consult with other doctors to come to a responsible conclusion. Remember, the doctor is seeing you because you are coming in with symptoms, not a diagnosis, and he must relate those symptoms to a cause. Doctors do not treat symptoms as much as the cause of those symptoms.

Finding a cause is not as simple as it may sound. As a matter of fact, we often go through the process of *ruling out* serious disorders, eventually reaching the point where we can tell you what you don't have, but we can't exactly tell you what you *do* have. This usually means that it probably is nothing serious and you can live with it for a while and it will probably go away. We don't have to do anything about it because if there is a change, you'll come back.

Because medicine is not an exact science, the doctor cannot diagnose and then treat a disorder simply by running a few tests and pushing a few buttons and returning you to your original health. This is frustrating not only to your doctor, but also to you as a pilot. You are used to immediate response to something going wrong. Your emergency checklist is prepared to consider every conceivable cause and to give you an immediate solution. Not so medicine. It can take days, weeks, or even months to thoroughly evaluate and treat your disorder. This is very difficult for the pilot to accept, and he is tempted by his equally anxious colleagues to take inappropriate courses of action. This understandable situation can only lead to a more difficult conclusion that eventually will have to be explained to the FAA.

In this process, we will often practice "defensive medicine," doing more tests than necessary and treating aggressively to cover our backsides from overlooking a rare disease or being accused of malpractice. The patient even expects this. Nevertheless, the doctor works towards a goal of diagnosis and therapy by first ruling out serious conditions, and then getting on with taking care of the *symptoms* (which you came in to see him for in the first place). In any case, the non-pilot patient can go back to work. If there is a change or if it doesn't get any better, he returns to the doctor. This is an ongoing, continuous process—of evaluation, ruling out and treatment until the symptoms go away or a more definitive diagnosis is made along with a specific, curative treatment. The difference between private and FAA practice is that the private doctor is trying to find the cause of the symptoms of an unhealthy person and population and then treat them; and the FAA is trying to prove the absence of disease in a usually healthy population.

This whole process is meant to keep you healthy, and if your own family doctor is comfortable with your health and his care, why doesn't this philosophy work for the FAA? The biggest difference is that the FAA looks at your health as something which should not change in the near future, usually one-to-two years from the time you are examined. The FAA knows full well that you will not come running to your AME if there is a change in your medical status. Therefore, the AME must determine, at the time of your physical, whether you have a medical problem or are likely to develop one. If you come in with symptoms that an AME finds potentially disqualifying, it must be determined that the data are not a problem for flying now or in the future. This determination requires a more extensive evaluation — probably more of an evaluation than your own doctor would find necessary. You are reluctant to divulge too much information for fear that something will turn up, and the doctor will be the first one to admit that if any doctor does enough tests on you, he is bound to find something wrong.

So what happens with these results? With the private, non-flying patient, the doctor will probably just observe for weeks and months.

Pilot's Manual of Medical Certification

The FAA, however, knows that it can't monitor you on a daily or weekly basis, so it requires more data to confirm that your present good health will remain. The evaluation necessary to provide these data may not be "medically justified." Therefore, you are caught between two types of medical evaluation standards: A set of results that could ground you, but standards that would be medically acceptable to your doctor. There is also a third standard—you yourself may not feel that the problem is disqualifying.

For most people, the tests the doctor uses and how he treats patients is the doctor's responsibility, and he will continue to take appropriate measures to keep the patient healthy. He is working without having to answer to anyone else but himself and his patients, certainly to no bureaucracy. Even if the process takes several weeks or months, the patient still can work. This may not be true for you as a pilot, however, since the FAA must assure that your disorder, the test results, and your therapy will not interfere with your flying responsibilities now and in the future, something your private doctor doesn't usually need to consider. Consequently, the FAA may require you to have more data to establish your present and potential health. Data your family doctor may not feel are required. Therefore, coupled with your doctor's defensive process, all this data may be more than is realistically necessary to keep your health, and usually in retrospect would not have been needed at all if you had known what to do to keep healthy.

You can now understand the dilemma. What your own doctor would do in your own best *medical* interests may not coincide with what the FAA needs, and you certainly don't want to be gounded. Your doctor may feel that your disorder is perfectly safe to fly with, yet if your doctor knew about flying, he'd know the disorder could be risky. By the same token, the FAA may accept a medical condition without a lot of extensive evaluation and treatment as long as it does not create a problem in the years to come. Also, the FAA may accept a disorder that your own doc wouldn't, especially if your doctor were somewhat afraid of flying. For example, the FAA will accept a blood pressure that would be too high in your own doctor's estimation. In contrast, as I stated earlier, the FAA may want more information than your own doctor feels is necessary. Remember, one of the tools that your family doctor can use is "tincture of time" and observation; the FAA must have immediate and current objective data with which to work and pass judgment on your flying status now and to anticipate the future. Your own doctor may feel that there is no reason why you can't fly, but your doctor probably doesn't know that your problem could be unsafe. I have seen many reports from well-meaning physicians stating that in *their* conclusion you, the patient, can fly, when in fact the problem is a severe threat to safety of flying. This is misleading to the unknowing pilot.

Thus, this triple standard: yours, your doctor's and the FAA's (and you could even add the additional standard of your colleagues).

As we discussed earlier, cardiovascular disease—high blood pressure and coronary artery disease—is one of the most common causes of medical groundings. In the case of increased blood pressure, medication is often the treatment of choice, but this treatment is also a direct threat to a pilot's career. Coronary artery disease is viewed by your doctor as treatable simply with observation, changing of lifestyle by developing an exercise program, losing weight, etc., and the use of medication to control any complications. To a pilot, however, merely the *history* of having significant coronary artery disease is a mandatory disqualification. If you have acquired this disorder, you are grounded.

So what's my point? If you are ill or notice symptoms which you haven't had before (assuming you are in excellent health to begin with), you must work *with* your family doctor so that in addition to caring for your health, he understands your minimum flying requirements. Be sure that he doesn't become overly aggressive in his evaluation or therapy, but does enough to obtain adequate information if the FAA requires it. Remember that your doctor probably knows little about the FAA and its procedures and probably even less about how your medical condition and the effects of this therapy on your ability to fly safely. He could be a "white knuckler" and overly protective about your flying health, or you may think that he is fully aware of the ramifications of the disorder on flying and allow you to continue flying when in the eyes of the FAA and a qualified aeromedical physician, your condition would not be compatible with safe flying. An interesting question is whether to tell a pilot too much despite wanting to keep him informed of his health. An analogy would be whether or not a pilot should tell his passengers that he has lost an engine, even though they are in no danger and they will not have to turn back. The passengers may expect to be informed, but is this information in the best interests of the passengers, especially if they don't understand? Therefore, be sure your doctor doesn't "tag" you in the record with too many "possible diagnoses." The record may come back to haunt you if not discretely defined. I am not advocating ignoring a medical problem or stating that it should not be corrected. But knowing that there is this dilemma, it is quite frustrating to me to realize that the majority of the medical disorders that ground a pilot could not only be corrected and controlled, but actually prevented if the pilot would follow common-sense health maintenance which I have discussed throughout this book, know the certification process and trust professional people. I realize that most pilots will not be concerned about their health until something goes wrong, but too many problems are created by waiting.

I would like to make a comment here regarding a relatively common feeling among some pilots in commercial aviation. There is a notion, especially among some of the "leaders" of the pilot community, that, "not only is the FAA out to get you—but so is the company." This is fortunately the exception, not the rule. However, this exception has been rumored enough within your environment to discredit the works of some company aviation doctors and dedicated private-practice aviation doctors who truly are on the pilot's side. The doctor must "play by the rules" of scientific, factual medicine. His critics, however, don't need to follow these rules because they are not responsible for your health and safety. A doctor can't necessarily resolve your problem in a matter of hours. This apparent inefficiency is not an indication of that doctor's worth. Whether you like the doctor and his results or not, he is still the only one who knows about your true health and he is only a messenger of the news, not the cause. Would you accept the comments of a friend over that of a professional mechanic when dealing with the health of your aircraft? Everybody loses if you don't fly, including the airline. To put the "doctor's out to get you" philosophy in a pilot's mind is unfair to the pilot who may want to look to that doctor for assistance in the future. With a career at stake, unfounded comments are an injustice to the worried pilot. At least check out the other side of the stories you hear. By understanding the philosophy that I am describing in this book, there is nothing lost by checking into your alternatives.

Usually if a pilot is medically grounded by the company doctor, aviation doctor or FAA, it is for a valid reason, a reason not often shared with the rest of the world. The outsiders pass judgment based upon what they hear: "Joe couldn't possibly be sick enough to ground—it must be the doc's screwing up." This, in my estimation, does a gross disservice to those of us who are trying to keep our flight crews flying. Remember, the doctor is only the messenger of that information that states you are not healthy. *You* are the one who has the abnormal condition, not the doc. The doc can't simply ignore it. There is, however, a way to keep control yourself. Find out about your health. Know about how the FAA works in certifying pilots, and keep healthy. Find an aeromedical physician who is knowledgeable—one that you can trust—then stick with him. You don't have to rely on rumors to guide you if *you* know what to expect. Keep ahead of your health and certification. That way you can avoid a premature report to the FAA.

Your challenge of protecting that medical certificate should now be clear—how to keep healthy, cure your illness (even though you rarely get sick), and hang onto your medical certificate without making waves with the FAA. Meeting this challenge is not that difficult, and, as I continue to stress, you *do* have control over your flying career.

Therefore, check up on your family doctor and AME. Do they really understand your requirements? Is the AME a pilot? What does the AME do with the medical reports—does he send them immediately to the FAA? How active is the AME in the professional organizations that promote knowledge in general medicine and aerospace medicine? I encourage *you* to become more familiar with the FAA's standards and procedures. Don't expect your family doctor to be thinking about you as a pilot or to understand that without a medical certificate you are permanently disabled from your job. You are still just a patient to him. Communicate this to your family doctor or trusted AME and actually work with the FAA to protect your certificate. This is not an easily accepted philosophy, but hear me out. If there still is doubt in your mind whether your own doctor is adequately evaluating or over-evaluating, or whether he is over-treating or under-treating, or if your health could affect your career, you might consider calling Oklahoma City or your regional FAA flight surgeon and, without using your name, ask for his advice. If you know of a knowledgeable AME or have an aeromedical consultant, call him. If you don't know an aeromedical doctor, then find one who is known and respected by the FAA. Recommendations from these doctors are considered very important in the FAA's mind. In addition, I am sure that your own doctor would be glad to know what to do or not to do since he is looking out for your future as well as for your health. If there is no reason to distrust your company aviation doctor or AME, keep him informed. He could be your strongest ally in protecting your medical certificate. He can't help you if you don't share with him how you are feeling and what is going on with your own family doctor. Of all the pilots who have used this philosophy, perhaps one percent have not benefited, but you won't hear about the 99 percent who *were* helped. That's not much incentive for a worried pilot to seek help. You must put your trust in somebody. With so much at stake—not only your health, but also your career—assume, unless you *know* or are sure otherwise, that the company doctor or aviation doc is truly on your side and is anxious to help you if you would allow him to do so.

If you still wish to see your own private doctor for maintaining your health and then your AME to get certified, that's fine. Just be sure that your private doctor knows about you as a pilot, and that your AME will cooperate if anything abnormal is found. What you learn in this book will be an adequate guide to help both. As I mentioned before, if there is any doubt about the status of your health, ground yourself, but seek help yourself from a competent AME or from the FAA anonymously. Don't depend upon aeromedically uninformed doctors who can create more problems. Check with those who truly know. Better still, keep ahead of everything by knowing the status of your health and by practicing a good health-maintenance program so you don't get caught behind the power curve.

To summarize what I have been saying, work with your family doctor (and then go to your AME if you wish), or, better still, work with an AME:

1. Know and understand the process of certification and how medical disorders affect your flying and consequently your certificate.
2. Find that AME or private doctor who has good credentials, is active in aviation and aviation medicine, and is willing to take the time and effort to work with you.
3. Judge this AME or private doctor by your own experience, not from hearsay or rumors from disgruntled pilots. Judge him by asking him about those subjects which we have discussed. Does he know what to do? Has he done it before, and what will he do if he finds something wrong? Does he know what additional information the FAA will need if a disorder is found?
4. If there is any doubt about your disorder being prematurely reported to the FAA, tell your doctor or AME that you will not fly. That is, you will ground yourself until the problem is resolved and a report to the FAA can be defered. A report to the FAA can then be made when *you* are ready.
5. Before your doctor puts you on medicine that you could be taking for an extended period, be sure that there are no other ways to control your problems such as diet, exercise, stress management, etc.
6. Show your doctor what your requirements are, and if you are skeptical, have him call the FAA or a professional aeromedical physician.
7. Take it upon yourself to practice good health maintenance so you don't get caught in the middle.
8. If you know of a problem that may be initially disqualifying, refer back to chapter three for the specifics on preserving your medical certificate.

Remember, the issue is, are you medically safe to fly? Your "ability" to fly unfortunately, has no bearing on your "fitness" to fly. You must accept that ultimate responsibility and you may have to "educate" your doctor and your AME.

6

A Pilot's Own Health Maintenance Program

A 46-year-old corporate pilot was overweight and out of shape and cared little about his "self image" and spent most of his free time in front of the TV. His wife was no example of an ideal spouse, either. Fortunately (or unfortunately), he could pass his FAA exam without problems and had little incentive to change his lifestyle. However, a grounded pilot did get his attention by spending some time explaining that he also did not take his health seriously and was suddenly grounded because of increased blood pressure. The pilot and his wife re-evaluated their priorities, and they both got back into shape and now actually enjoy their free time.

LOOK BACK AT WHEN you were introduced to IFR flying, and you watched with awe at how easily and rewarding it was for the "real" pilot to break out of the clouds with the runway approach lights right down the middle. And then *you* began an attempt at putting it all together. You quickly found that flying an aircraft was one thing, but flying the gauges, communicating with ATC, and reading approach plates added a seemingly overwhelming burden to even the most professional pilot. But you finally got it together and you realized that most of what you now were doing—flying IFR—was by habit. You didn't have to think out everything that you had to do. How did this learning happen?

If you recall, you first read books. Then you had someone show you how IFR works, and then you practiced what you read and were shown. And you continue to do this to this day. The proof of your success is passing the periodic check ride.

Developing your own health-maintenance program is similar. You can't expect to do the job without preparation any more than you can learn to fly the ILS back-course by only watching your instructor. You can't just listen to your doctor and assume that the job will get done — he has no magic pills; nor can you put your career in his hands and expect him to get you out of trouble that you brought about yourself with abuses to your health.

So the first thing you must do is *know the regulations* that concern your health. You can't assume that the doctor knows these regulations any more or less than you.

Then you must learn your *true* health status by having a good medical evaluation with a doctor who knows the rules. Some will say that the periodic complete physical is overdone and, in the general public, it might be. But a professional pilot not only must be healthy when he's at the controls, he must protect his career by staying healthy. He must take the physicals to keep ahead. Ideally, he should have a medical "preflight" exam every time he flies, but that's totally unrealistic and couldn't be done in the best interests of the *pilot*. Yet, it should be the same philosophy as in preventive maintenance of aircraft. Just like in your dual training, this evaluation must be with someone you can trust and respect. This must be someone who will do the job right the first time and not feel that he has to personally run to the FAA if you can't get it right the first time.

The evaluation should include a thorough physical exam, a chest x-ray, a *resting* EKG, blood and urine tests, breathing tests, a test for blood in your bowel movements, and the usual vision and hearing tests. The most *important* part of any medical evaluation is a comprehensive, candid, yet confidential medical history. This history rarely is shared with a doctor except with the most trusted physicians — usually not AMEs. It still remains that this history is vitally important for the doctor in order for him to fully evaluate you.

From this evaluation, you determine your risk factors, factors that could statistically decrease your chances of keeping your medical certificate. You can't improve or correct faults that lead to increased risk until you identify them. What is your cholesterol level? Has your EKG changed? Are you overweight and out of shape? Once you have identified your risk factors (or confirmation of good health), you can begin to practice correcting them, and practice, and practice, until you are sure that you can pass your next physical without fear and you have developed good health *habits*.

By identifying your risk factors and trying to correct them, you begin to determine what factors keep you from achieving your goal — your perfect "medical check ride." Is it habit and lack of self-control or is it too much temptation that keeps those risk factors ever present — you have been trying haven't you? So how do you improve that over-correcting tendency on the glide slope? It's the same technique of learning good health *habits* — practice and patience. There is no short cut to health maintenance or to maintaining flying proficiency.

It is all well and good to identify your problems, and I am sure you have tried many times to correct those risk factors, but it still doesn't work. Why? You certainly are motivated. You really know what has to be done, but it just doesn't progress the way the books say. You continue to gain weight and you still smoke too much, and you rationalize that "as long as I feel good—not to worry." But you do when you take your FAA exam.

The solution should be apparent. You can't do it alone, and *you can't do it without changing old habits first.* That means working with your doctor and his assistants, giving them time to explain what needs to be done, and then practicing and returning, practicing and returning, practicing and returning. You may have to guide the "doc" on what *your* special aeromedical needs are, but *he* knows the medical part. Find out what the "ideal" healthy pilot should be. Talk to others who have licked the same problem. Don't depend upon techniques that are not generally accepted. Get the facts. Stick to your plan, but remember that few people have been able to do it alone. A pilot's pride is no less than a doctor's, and I know it is hard for doctors to let go of old ideas and lifestyles and change to new ones. Our egos get in the way of logical health maintenance. Remember, though, I can go back to work with an illness.

When considering claims for a "new and revolutionary" diet or health-maintenance program, which may not be generally accepted or proven useful by the medical profession, remember that a promoter of this program is not obligated to discuss the pros and cons. The doctor, on the other hand, must advise you of his recommendations; after all, he ultimately is responsible for your health. He can do this only after considering all sides of the issue, and his advice must be tailored to your individual requirements. In other words, if John Doe advertises his new program for better health, he will use *only* those studies and testimonials which will further *his* cause. He will not use any reports that could dispute his claim. Now, if *Doctor* John Doe or your own doctor is asked what he thinks of a particular program, he is obligated, in your best interest, to share all sides of the claimed benefits. This results in an inherent impression of negativism on the part of the doctor, which adds to the frustration of the pilot looking for a good program. What to do? Consider the source, his experience, and whether or not he considers the "cons" as well as the "pros." No program is free of these "cons." Look more to your own doctor for advice. Don't play doctor. Your family and friends are poor medical consultants.

I once had an instrument instructor who gave me some simple, but wise, advice: If the job needs doing, do whatever it takes to get the job done. We all are inherently impatient and want to see objective results

Pilot's Manual of Medical Certification

_____'s
Health Maintenance
PROGRESS

Date Began _____   Beginning Weight _____

Who Committed To: Beginning Pulse _____

_____   Beginning Blood Pressure

_____

GOALS:

• PULSE
■ WEIGHT

3 month weight _____

3 month pulse _____

6 month weight _____

6 month pulse _____

in a matter of days or weeks. When we don't see the change right away, we become discouraged and slip back into our old, comfortable, unchallenging habits. The job doesn't get done by simply studying the problem and not taking action.

You now know what is expected of you by the FAA. You also are —or should be—working with a doctor who knows your health and recognizes the limitations put on you by the FAA and your flying responsibilities. As a result, you have identified your risk factors and have made an attempt to identify the elements controlling them. For example, you are overweight and your cholesterol and triglycerides are up. You have recorded your intake in a good diary so you know where the extra calories and fatty foods are coming from. You talk with your spouse and discuss how the meals can be modified to correct the problem. But what about when you are on a trip? Those flight lunches leave a lot to be desired. What do you order when you go out to eat? Go back to the basics described in the chapter on eating. Who says you can't "brown bag" your meals? Who says you have to clean your plate?

But the motivation will get weaker unless you really have changed that old lifestyle. This gets us into the hardest part: how to maintain the drive that keeps everything under control.

Try different tricks. Tack a copy of your medical certificate and the above form on the refrigerator door or on the mirror in the bathroom to remind you to eat right and to start exercises. Fill in the blanks on this progress sheet and monitor the results of your efforts. Get a buddy with the same problem and support each other. Return to your doctor's office to check-in for monitoring. Sure it is expensive and a nuisance—but it beats sitting at home grounded.

The key to the success of your health-maintenance program is knowing what has to be done and why, and working with someone who can be very objective with your program, so let's review the steps:

1. Know your obligations and restrictions by being familiar with the FAR Part 67.

2. Fully understand and be comfortable with the meaning of FAR 61.53, especially the strategy of not immediately reporting to the FAA.

3. Know your *true* health and identify risk factors by having a periodic, *thorough* medical evaluation by a doctor who knows your requirements and restrictions.

4. Under the supervision of your doctor, change your old habits and learn healthier habits.

5. If there is any doubt about your doctor's knowledge about *your* obligations to the FAA, teach him. Be sure your doctor or his assis-

tants are willing and able to help you in your ongoing health-maintenance program.

6. Finally, keep on top of your health status, just as you do with your flying status. Keep working at your goals. If one way doesn't work, try another. "Do whatever it takes to get the job done." Monitor yourself continuously and have someone "keep score" for you.

This monitoring need not require fancy tests or frequent returns to your doctor or therapist. Measurements *you* can take and *record* will be an excellent guide to how you are progressing. These include how your clothes fit, your pulse rate at rest and with exercise, your weight, the measurement of your waist and biceps, how you are sleeping (are you rested in the morning?), what belt holes are you using (hang your belt up everynight so you can see it). You might even consider taking a picture of yourself once a month for comparison.

Earlier in the book, I expressed my feelings about the "pass the buck" philosophy of some AMEs. This philosophy also can pertain to you because many pilots who fail at health maintenance want to blame someone else. A favorite "cover your rear end" statement by people promoting a new diet or health aid that may not work is "ask your doctor." Well, he can't help you either if you don't watch your lifestyle. If you approach a health maintenance program as you would when "cramming for an exam," then not continue good health maintenance practices, you are jeopardizing your career, even though you passed the test. Anyone can pass an exam by cramming.

Unfortunately, many professional pilots have much of their flying career spelled out for them (FARs, company policies, etc.), and some have a lot of the mundane parts of flying done for them (filing flight plans, obtaining weather reports, etc.). This allows the pilot to concentrate on flying, but it also gives him a false sense of "who is responsible" in other matters dealing with his career, especially his medical certificate. I hope that by now you will realize no one is watching your health. Only you are responsible for it. The FAA and your company are looking for the unhealthy, but *you* are responsible for not being one of those who allowed their poor health to interfere with their career.

Unlike most other aspects of professional flying, your medical status and how you maintain good health are purely up to you. You picked a career that required good health and also the requirement of proof of that good health to a government agency. By staying healthy and understanding the certification process, there is very little chance of your being unnecessarily grounded. I have stated it many times, and I will state it once more. Don't let the FAA be the one to get your attention to do the things you should be doing anyway to remain a healthy and safe pilot. Plan on reaching retirement—healthy.

7

Airworthy Anatomy
by
SHARON M. HANKS

A 43 year old airline pilot had a problem with weight. He just couldn't loose more than a few pounds without gaining them back. Over the years, his blood pressure continued to rise. He became a "ping-pong dieter", going on crash diets prior to his FAA exam and then allowing the fat to return. Eventually, his blood pressure reached a consistently elevated state regardless of his weight. He's flying, but he's under constant monitoring by the FAA even though he finally got his weight under control.

EVEN UNDER A DELUGE of duties, demands, decisions and dangers, a pilot is expected to function with optimum efficiency at all times.

The level of responsibility involved in expertly maneuvering a massive airplane around our world and safely transporting thousands of precious lives is very high—it requires the pilot to function without error. He must exhibit utmost mental capability, extreme emotional stability and excellent physical condition to meet the superhuman expectations.

Certainly, you would expect that a pilot would do absolutely everything in his power to safeguard the workings of his intricate human machine, for his very career depends upon the premise of good health. But it seems as though pilots often give more attention to the "health" of their aircraft than to the health of their bodies. Pilots would never consider going on a trip without having enough fuel aboard their airplanes, but, ironically, they are willing to begin the day's journey without enough fuel in their bodies—without having eaten an adequate breakfast. The pilot knows that it would be foolish to expect a 747 to execute a successful take-off burning gasohol, and yet at times he tries to squeeze his essential minimum daily requirements out of a dozen cups of coffee. He also seeks to prevent any possible mechanical failure by conducting a thorough preflight while, in contrast, his own bodily "gauges" and "indicators" of impending physical failure go unnoticed or disregarded. In reality, however, even the mighty pilot is not immune to human shortcomings of improper eating and activities that can have devastating effects on maintaining his airworthy anatomy and his career.

Eating sensibly is vital to maintaining excellent health and physical fitness. This applies to everyone: young, old, male, female, rich and poor. You probably have heard the phrase, "you are what you eat." Obviously, what you are is not limited only to what you eat. What you are as a person also is influenced by what you see, what you hear, what you read, what you know, what you experience, etc. But speaking in terms of physical body, the tangible, what you are is, most accurately, what goes down the hatch. That rich, red blood that rushes in tiny rivulets to the far reaches of the body, hastening the emergency oxygen rations to deficient, suffocating cells when you soar at high altitudes . . . those sturdy bones comprising your frame that support your movements and allow you to board and operate the aircraft . . . those delicate brain cells that miraculously spark every instantaneous thought, every crucial cockpit calculation . . . all of these, and virtually every single cell of your body, are formed and maintained by using the vital substances gleaned from the foods—or "unfoods"—that you eat. The importance of the quality of your food should be quite obvious. But, in spite of the apparent significance, getting all of the proper kind of food fuel for the body, in the correct amounts, all too often is overlooked.

The problems associated with food and nutrition are very different today than they were years ago. The problem for man in the past was to provide enough food for himself and his family for subsistence. Man had to battle nature to grow his own crops and raise his own livestock. He suffered from all kinds of dietary deficiencies and natural diseases. In contrast, food and nutrition problems in the United States today are just the opposite. Food is overly abundant, available and appealing. Our problem is eating too much, and yet too poorly for a well-balanced diet. No longer do we "eat to live" but the emphasis is now becoming "live to eat." No longer do we struggle to satisfy hunger, but instead we indulge the appetite. It is estimated that 30-50 percent of the population of the United States is obese.

By the way, chubby, the term obese does not only apply to the "other guy" at whom you are pointing a finger, but it includes such states as being "pleasingly plump," "roly-poly," and "slightly overweight," terms that are used to make light of a seriously heavy situation. We continue to eat ourselves to death, literally. It has become a way of life.

Ironically, at the same time that Americans boast of technological accomplishments, advancements in medical science, great strides in food production and an ever-increasing knowledge of nutrition, this country is faced with epidemic proportions of nutritionally related degenerative diseases like heart disease, atherosclerosis, hypertension, stroke, diabetes, obesity and anemias. We are proud because we are so rich and food is so abundant, but heart disease continues to be our number one killer. We consume a disproportionate percentage of the world's available foodstuffs while trying—unsuccessfully—to ignore the consequences of being overweight. We hardly know the meaning of scarcity, starvation or famine. Some countries don't know the meaning of heart disease, atherosclerosis and obesity!

The abuse of food accompanied by the neglect of physical activity has placed us in the midst of a coronary epidemic, where we are forced to deal with diseases that we can't blame on the invasion of microorganisms. We can't pass the buck to infection by innocent bacteria or viruses. Instead, we have brought a plague upon ourselves by our own mistakes, apathy, affluence and unwillingness to listen to the advice of those who are trying desperately to help. People are always willing to listen and change their ways after having had a heart attack—provided they survive it. It is unfortunate that it takes such drastic and painful measures to arouse their interest. It is especially disastrous for the pilot, who not only jeopardizes his health but also loses his cherished career in the process.

The American lifestyle, verging on gluttony, condones very rich foods and empty calories in infinite quantities, in conjunction with a dangerously reduced activity level. Our consumption of the fat-laden meats and dairy products has been on the rise while there has been a noticeable trend of diminished purchasing of the valuable, vitamin-rich fruits, vegetables and grains. Our frenzied pace has encouraged more frequent use of restaurants, especially the fast-food type. We also are relying more on heavily processed junk foods. Hard physical labor has given way to sedentary desk work. Driving has replaced that valuable means of transportation, walking. The use of leisure time in recreation and sports has been undermined by the art of gawking motionlessly at the "tube" for hours on end, with all-too-frequent trips to the refrigerator.

The eventual consequences of all of this physical idleness and overeating to our heart's content—or more accurately, at our heart's expense—are unavoidable. If not brought under control these bad habits soon can force one to become a mere statistic in the national mortality tables. Fortunately, you *can* employ a better lifestyle, one of prudent eating and exercise, and work toward the prevention of heart disease. You *can* reduce your risk of heart disease and its associated diseases, and possibly even reverse the degenerative process to some extent. So don't just sit back like a timebomb ready to explode and wait for some warning. By the time symptoms of heart disease appear the insidious illness has already progressed far. Sometimes the fatal heart attack is the first and final warning! And then no physician's good intentions, no miracle drug, no magic wand, no sum of money, no amount of fame, can mend that neglected heart. The time to act is now, just when you think you don't need to act.

Every human being has the instinct to survive, that internal drive to live. We all have the desire and the right to a long, healthy and happy life. Our bodies are supposed to last—they were made that way—to be strong and not break down during prime years. It was not intended that high blood pressure, diabetes, stroke and heart problems prematurely halt your most productive years. Pilots are supposed to reach 60 and well beyond. Unlike some other machines, the human machine improves with use. Inactivity only causes degradation. Sensible eating, accompanied by vigorous physical activity, is essential to optimal health and longevity. This is no big surprise. So why do so many people still face serious health problems?

Health has received a great deal of public attention in recent years. Nutritional controversies saturate the media, causing much confusion. You undoubtedly have been bombarded with articles about nutritional cults, food faddists, "miracle" diets, the harmful effects of table sugar, cholesterol and heart disease, additives and preservatives, yogurt as a "cure-all," health food stores, megavitamins, and many, many more issues. Further complicating the matter is the power of Madison Avenue ads capable of selling any product, good or bad. The health food/weight loss business is a multimillion-dollar industry preying on you and me, making it very difficult to know the truth about sensible eating. It is my intention to weed through the cluttered media mess for you in order to salvage some facts.

Actually, some of the very basic rules of a good, sound diet have not changed much over the years. Their age does not make them invalid, just as popularity does not guarantee credibility. Therefore, don't be too quick to discard rules that you learned years ago and latch onto every new idea that comes along. Instead, be informed and wise in discerning the beneficial suggestions from the useless or harmful. Incorporate new findings gradually and intelligently so that the important ideas become a permanent part of your life and not merely a brief fling.

THE FUEL

When it comes to eating, why do you choose that substance commonly known as food? Why not have a bowl of gravel with a side order of wood shavings to get your minerals and fiber?

The main reason for eating a meal in the first place is to consume the foods that contain all of the necessary ingredients to provide the cells of the body with the supplies for energy, building and repair. This is your main thought while perusing a menu of delectables in your favorite French restaurant, right? Ridiculous! For man, the act of eating has become more complex. If procuring nutrients were the only consideration in the formation of our dining habits, our procedure could be quite primitive. We might just as well drag ourselves up next to the nearest fuel tank, snap on a hose to the ol' stomach, and proceed to "fill 'er up." It would be an uncomplicated, mechanical maneuver, just like fueling your aircraft or gassing your car. No decision, no selection, no recipe preparation, no mess, no time, no waste — just pump it in until the gauges indicate "enough."

Fortunately, but unfortunately for some abusers, eating has become a much more complex, civilized activity. Eating is a pleasurable, satisfying experience. Food entices the senses with visual appeal, savory aromas, assorted textures and a spectrum of flavors. Mealtime is an important part of home life and family togetherness. Eating is a pleasant part of daily living around which many social and business gatherings are planned. Eating habits have cultural qualities and great national diversity. Some foods have deep religious symbolism. All of our cherished holidays and traditions are intertwined with foods of particular significance. Even the changing seasons influence our eating; we anticipate the revival of certain foods that make their limited annual appearance. Consider also the phenomenon called munching, a casual perversion of conscious intelligent ingestion, that goes hand-in-hand, or hand-to-mouth, with spectator sports and movies. These are only a few of the many factors that contribute to the intricacies of our eating habits.

Obviously, our selection of foods should be based largely on the actual content of the product and how it benefits the body. But many subconscious factors negatively influence our decisions and may jeopardize our health. It is important to be knowledgeable about food facts while being aware of the outside forces, both good and bad, in order to remain in control of your intake.

We're talking about food. So what is food, anyway? Take a moment to scrutinize it. See that buffet table heaped with beautifully prepared gourmet delights, colorful arrangements of luscious chef's masterpieces, and exquisite, rare delicacies? A gorgeous sight . . . better than crew meals! Try to think about needs for a moment instead of wants, as impossible as that seems in this situation. Remember that there is more to food than tastes, smells, and a distended abdomen. Nutrition is the process by which the substances that you eat *become YOU.* What you eat today flies the plane tomorrow! The nutrient part of that food is really what your body is seeking. And you can find it even at the smorgäsbord if you look past the frills and embellishments, around the garnishes and decorations, and through the marinades and sauces. Food is dressed up and camouflaged with infinite variety, but if you zoom in for a microscopic view you find that each dish consists of the same, common, minute building blocks called nutrients. Everything from the Chateaubriand to the chocolate mousse can be broken down into six essential kinds of nutrients—proteins, carbohydrates, fats, vitamins, minerals and water. Stack the building blocks one way and you have a pork chop. Stack 'em another way and you've got a string bean.

Nutrients are actually chemical substances, arrangements of atoms into complex molecules, naturally occurring in foods, that work together and interact with body chemicals. They are essential for building, operation and repair of body tissue, for efficient functioning, and for furnishing fuel. Each nutrient has a specific use in the body. No one natural food, by itself, contains all the required nutrients. Many kinds and combinations of foods together can lead to a well-balanced diet. Therefore, you need a variety of foods each day to assure that you are getting all the different, necessary nutrients. Everyone needs the same nutrients throughout life but in different amounts depending on age, sex, activity level, occupation, environmental stress, size, state of health, pregnancy, etc.

Every single bite that you take at each meal and in between, has to be processed by your body, and has an effect in the body immediately and cumulatively. Your body has to deal with every particle of that delicious T-bone that you had last night while on layover, as well as every additive in that sleezy hotdog that you just "inhaled" during the last brief stop. Don't think that you can eat something just for the fun of it and that it then will simply pass right through you and out. Having a piece of pie à la mode after a huge banquet doesn't mean that the pie won't have any effect on the way through the system. Something has to be done with it, even though you didn't *need* it. Your body either will use it or store it (and you know where) along with the extras from yesterday . . . and the day before . . . and the day before that. Sorry. Get the picture?

Long after you chow down, your digestive system is hard at work processing the food and breaking it down into nutrients or nutrient combinations and waste products. The blood which is continually circulating absorbs nutrients from the digestive tract and oxygen from the lungs, and carries them to each cell in the body. Some of the essential nutrients need to be replenished every day. Others can be stored for future use, but an excess of one never can compensate for a shortage of another. Sometimes certain nutrients are only effective when working together as "teams." For example, in building bones, the nutrients vitamin D, calcium and phosphorus must interact. One member of the team cannot perform its job unless all the others are present in the right proportions. Thus, variety of foods and moderation in amount are two key concepts in a wise eating pattern.

Protein

Protein is required by all living things. It is the basic substance making up every cell of the body and is needed by everyone throughout life for many important functions:
- Building and maintaining body tissues
- Rapid tissue growth during childhood, pregnancy
- After excess destruction or loss, such as burns, surgery, hemorrhage, infection
- Making hemoglobin which carries oxygen to the cells and carbon dioxide away from the cells
- Making up part of the DNA molecule that carries the genetic code
- Production of thousands of enzymes, which control the chemical reactions of the body
- Production of hormones, which regulate body processes
- Supplying energy in shortage situations
- Regulating water balance and the acid-base balance

Protein is made up of smaller chemical units called amino acids. During digestion the proteins from foods are broken down into amino acids, which are then rearranged into different proteins for special functions in the human body. There are 20 or more different amino acids, which serve as building blocks of proteins. The protein molecules resemble long chains where each link is an amino acid chemically joined by peptide bonds. Each protein molecule has hundreds of amino acids linked into long chains in an endless number of combinations and sequences, making possible an almost infinite variety of proteins.

The body can synthesize most of the amino acids from foods, but some must be provided ready-made in the diet. They are known as "essential" amino acids. There are eight: lysine, tryptophan, methionine, phenylalanine, threonine, valine, leucine and isoleucine. Food proteins providing all of the essential amino acids in the amounts and proportions needed by the body are known as "complete" proteins and rate highest in quality value. A low-value protein lacks one or more of the indispensable amino acids and cannot support life by itself. However, two different proteins with limiting amino acids may complement each other and together provide a higher value.

Animal products—meat, fish, poultry, milk, cheese and eggs—are high-quality proteins and are sources of readily available essential amino acids. Animal body composition is similar to that of humans and thus animal proteins supply more of the essential amino acids than plant foods. Fruits, vegetables, legumes and grains are lower in quality because some amino acids are missing. Higher quality protein foods can be teamed with lower quality protein foods to provide good total protein nutrition when eaten together. The missing amino acids can be "filled-in" to improve the overall balance. Some examples of "teams" are breakfast cereal with milk, rice with fish, macaroni with cheese, and spaghetti with meat sauce.

Some nutrients can be stored in the body for later use but protein cannot. It must be supplied in the diet every day. It is best used when consumed in small amounts every few hours. Protein deficiency is not a major problem today in the United States. In fact, most Americans eat much more protein than they need. This is biologically and economically wasteful. But Americans like lots of meat, and since they can afford to, they continue to consume large quantities of it, especially beef and pork. Years ago we used to rely heavily on the vegetable and grain sources of protein, but today the majority of our protein is taken from the more-expensive animal sources. We have decreased the consumption of vegetables and grains at the expense of losing some valuable substances, while our increased use of animal products, which are heavy with fats, has contributed to new health problems.

Some people still believe that they can only get "fat" around the middle from eating too many carbohydrates or too many food fats. But too many proteins can do the same thing. When burned, the carbohydrates and food fats supply most of the body's energy. When not enough calories are available from the carbohydrates and fats to meet the energy demand, *then* the body may use some of the extra free proteins for energy calories. But usually, excess proteins are converted to body fat. So you can actually become fat from eating excess calories in the protein form just as you can from eating too many carbohydrate calories or too many food-fat calories. It is the *surplus of calories* that adds pounds, regardless of where they came from. Overindulging in top quality steak can add inches to the waistline just as well as too many gooey sweet rolls.

Another misconception about proteins is that great quantities are needed to build muscle mass and to better one's athletic performance. Since meat is muscle, many coaches and athletes have believed that eating meat, especially red meat, would increase muscle mass and overall strength. Thick steaks have been approved for many training meals in the world of sports. Actually, only a small amount of additional protein is needed during athletic conditioning for developing muscles, and, as stated earlier, any excess protein is converted to body f-a-t. Eating a 16-ounce piece of beef does not mean that you would add ounces to your biceps, any more than eating hair would diminish a bald spot or eating brain would increase your smarts.

If you are disappointed in the image ridiculing you in the mirror, and you long for a Superman physique with the power of a locomotive, don't start investing in magical protein-supplement concoctions. The key to having the strong, bulging muscles is not in consuming a mountain of protein but in doing a heap of exercise. Standing around in telephone booths waiting for the Clark-Kent-metamorphic-zap is futile. Standing around, mild-mannered or not, never did anyone any good. You've got to get out and "move-it," man. If your goal is to be muscle-bound, a well-planned, supervised program of exercise, especially the isometrics and the isotonics, will bring the desired dimensions. Because of an increased energy expenditure while exercising, extra calories will be needed. They should come from a balanced diet emphasizing carbohydrates and fats, not extra protein. It is the exercise that induces muscle strength and hypertrophy, not more protein. We cannot make more muscle fibers in our bodies—the number stays the same—but we can force the ones that we have to get bigger.

Before you get too entangled in your vanity, keep in mind that exercise for the sole purpose of building the skeletal muscles is fine, and harmless to a certain extent. But all too often the one most-important and vital muscle in the whole body, the heart, is neglected. "Pumping iron" does build muscle mass for outward appearance, but it does nothing inside for your heart muscle. The additional muscle weight may even be a strain on the heart because of the increased mass that the heart must accommodate and also some vascular constriction may occur. Being muscle bound is purely aesthetic and has no real lasting purpose unless the heart is equally conditioned. Certain types of exercise do focus on strengthening the heart and greatly benefit your life in terms of overall health, physical endurance, and longevity. They are aerobic exercises such as running, bicycling, swimming, and walking. It is the cardiovascular system that needs the attention; we don't seem to be dying from weak arms, but weak hearts. You'll often find that the little, skinny guy who rides his bicycle to work every day has more cardiovascular endurance than Mr. Muscle, when put to a real test.

Carbohydrates

Carbohydrates are chemical combinations of carbon, hydrogen and oxygen.

In order to survive, all animals must eat plants that supply carbohydrates. Only plants contain chlorophyll, which enables them to make carbohydrates from the carbon dioxide in the air and water in the soil, while using the energy from the sun. Plant foods provide carbohydrates in three main forms: starches, sugars and celluloses (fiber).

Like proteins, carbohydrate molecules also resemble chains in structure, where each link is a sugar molecule. This is not the white sugar that you find on the kitchen table. A larger carbohydrate molecule, like starch, is a chain of the smaller simpler sugars as building blocks. All carbohydrates must be broken down by digestion into simple sugars to be used as a source of energy by body tissues. Glucose, commonly known as "blood sugar," is the form mainly used by the body's cells. Some complex carbohydrates, such as cellulose, cannot be broken down by digestion in man, and when eaten they simply supply the roughage that is needed for proper elimination of solid wastes.

The major function of carbohydrates in the body is to furnish the fuel for energy to do work, whether it be the silent, ongoing, internal body processes or all-out physical exertion. Glucose is one of the most important fuels. It is the main source of energy for red blood cells and the central nervous system—your brain!

Carbohydrates spare proteins from being used up for energy by fulfilling the energy needs themselves, and thus saving proteins for more important jobs such as tissue building and repair. Carbohydrates also help in the use of fats.

The body draws energy from carbohydrates mainly by converting the simple glucose molecule to carbon dioxide and water. This is one of the most vital chemical reactions in biology. It is the very essence of transforming the starch from a wonderfully nutritious baked potato (not just some oversweet bakery "fluff") into the actual energy needed to win a tennis match, fly an airplane, or just sit and breathe.

When there is more glucose in the body than can be used for energy, small amounts of the excess can be stored in the liver and muscles as glycogen, a starchy substance also referred to as "animal starch." But for the most part, the carbohydrates eaten in excess of the body's energy needs are quickly converted to body F-A-T. So, you can become overweight by eating too many calories in the carbohydrate form. But this is also true of excess protein calories and excess fat calories. Carbohydrates are *not* more "fattening" than the other two main nutrients. Excess calories in *any* form will add extra baggage for you to haul around.

It is a common misconception that carbohydrates, especially the starches, are more fattening than other foods. In so thinking people have avoided breads, potatoes and rice in an attempt to lose weight. How ridiculous! A gram of carbohydrate yields four calories. A gram of protein yields the same: four calories per gram. But for fats it is more than double: nine calories per gram. Ironically, a reduction in the quantity of carbohydrates in the diet usually results in eating more proteins which are usually accompanied by *fat*. This produces the opposite of the desired results by actually increasing the total calorie intake. Calories *do* count! Approximately 3,500 extra calories results in a pound. Its not complicated — just simple arithmetic.

The major carbohydrate sources are grains (corn, rice, wheat, oats), products made from grains (flour, bread, breakfast cereal, spaghetti, noodles, macaroni, grits), potatoes, dry beans and peas, tapioca, sugar beets and sugar cane. Most of the other fruits and vegetables have smaller amounts of carbohydrates. In vegetables it is chiefly in the starch form. In fruits it is mainly sugars.

Carbohydrates on the whole are very economical to produce in large quantities — a fact that the majority of the people in the world depend on for survival. Many countries rely on bread, potatoes, or rice to sustain their populations. Americans draw about half their total calories from carbohydrates, but of these, too many calories are consumed as white table sugar, soft drinks, cakes, candy and processed food. We're getting too many empty calories in forms that are deficient in vitamins and minerals and have detrimental side effects.

Sugar is used to flavor many foods and to provide quick energy. But foods high in sugar (sucrose) are high in calories and low in nutrient content. Refined sugar is an atypical "food" because it is pure carbohydrate . . . or pure calories. It has no protein, fat, vatamins or minerals. Most other foods contain combinations of the valuable nutrients, but not sugar. It is empty. What's worse, these "empty" calories tend to dull the appetite, further decreasing the intake of the *valuable* nutrients.

Sugars should only be eaten in moderation, but in the United States sugar consumption has been abused, and the level has reached about 100 pounds per person per year! This is because we are eating more concentrated sources of sugars as sweet manufactured products, huge quantities of soft drinks, bakery goods, cakes and candy, syrups, jams and jellies. This all contributes to our high incidence of obesity and diabetes.

Food qualities usually are described in terms of proteins, carbohydrates, fats, vitamins and minerals. A unique substance called fiber, or sometimes roughage, actually is a carbohydrate and should be included in our discussion here. Even though it is not absorbed by the body it does play a significant role in the digestive process.

Many fresh fruits, raw and cooked vegetables and whole grain cereals supply us with what we call bulk or roughage. The more popular term today is fiber. Fiber is the stiff, woody part of plants that support, coat or protect plant cells. It is composed of complex carbohydrates such as cellulose. For the most part, fiber is undigested as it goes through the digestive system but it has some beneficial effects on the way. As the unused food mass passes through the intestines, fiber helps to make the stool softer and bulkier to speed passage and aid regularity. Fiber also may increase the elimination of bile acids, sterols and fats. Scientists are studying other possible benefits of fiber in relation to disease prevention. One possible benefit is in preventing cancer of the colon.

The American eating style, with its de-emphasis on fruits, vegetables, grains, dried peas and beans, has tended toward less and less fiber content. Consumption of meat and dairy products, which do not provide fiber, has increased. A conscious effort is needed to stress those foods high in fiber.

Fats

Fats in our food have a variety of functions. As one of the three basic components of our food, fat is a very concentrated source of energy which can be used for all types of work and body processes. Gram for gram, fat yields more than twice as much energy when metabolized than either protein or carbohydrates. And if those extra calories are not used for energy, then they will be applied to fat deposits, or adipose tissue found just beneath the skin. Once again, the rule applies in that excess calories put the unwanted pounds on the body no matter whether they come from protein, carbohydrates or fat. Calories *do* count.

Some fat deposits are beneficial. A certain amount of fat in the tissues helps to cushion the vital organs for added protection against traumatic injury. Some fat deposits in the body serve as a sort of insulation to aid in maintaining proper body temperature. This type of insulation should not be confused with the present day home-insulation mania. In some instances where a little of something is good, a lot is better, like in insulating your attic. But this does not apply to the accumulation of body fat. Remember moderation? We don't condone the "tires" around your middle in terms of an increase in "R" value. Too much fat deposited in the body not only makes one overweight and unbecoming, but also disrupts all other body functions and can lead to serious, complicated health problems. What a price to pay!

Supplying energy is the primary function of fat and in this way it helps the body use protein and carbohydrates more efficiently for other purposes. But there are several other functions, too. Fats carry the fat-soluable vitamines—A,D,E and K—which are all essential. Fats also aid in the actual absorption of these vitamins. Fats add flavor and variety of texture to many of our foods. They can give you a satisfied feeling because they are digested slowly and delay the stimulation of a hunger sensation. Certain fats must be included in the diet to provide the body with linoleic acid, an essential fatty acid that the body cannot synthesize on its own. Linoleic acid is indispensible for life. It is necessary for growth, reproduction and healthy skin. You can find it especially in vegetable oils like corn, cottonseed, safflower, sesame, soybean, and wheat germ. It is also found in some nuts, poultry and fish.

The most common fats found in our food are known as triglycerides. As the name implies, they are chemically composed of three fatty acids plus one glycerol, which is an alcohol. As dietary fats are digested they are broken down into fatty acids and glycerol, the smaller building blocks. They are used by the body in this simpler form.

Nutritionists classify fatty acids in three categories: saturated, monounsaturated, and polyunsaturated, as TV commercials affirm. The names may sound complicated but their meanings really are simple. Each fatty acid is composed of carbon atoms joined like a chain, with as many as 20 carbons linked together. Every carbon atom has as many hydrogen atoms attached to it as it can hold. Like a sponge that is saturated with water and cannot absorb another drop, a *saturated* fatty acid contains the maximum number of hydrogens that it can hold. The unsaturated fatty acids, whether mono- or poly-, have some hydrogens missing from the molecule. A *monounsaturated* fatty acid has one location where hydrogen is missing and carbons have double bonded to each other instead. A *polyunsaturate* has two or more locations where hydrogens are missing in the same fashion. These terms simply refer to the chemical structure of the molecules. But you have heard them used more often in reference to their physical and dietary differences.

One of the differences between saturated and unsaturated fatty acids is in their physical properties. Saturated fats are usually solid at room temperature and are composed of longer carbon chains. Unsaturated fats are usually liquid at room temperature and are composed of shorter chains. Although all of the fats, whether from plant or animal sources, are composed of a combination of both saturated and unsaturated fatty acids, the fats from animal sources such as butter, lard, or bacon generally are more saturated and solid at room temperature than the vegetable sources, like the liquid polyunsaturated vegetable oils. Of course, there are exceptions and variations within each group. For instance, in the meat group, beef and pork are much higher in saturated fats than poultry and fish, even though they all are from animal sources. The degree of saturation also may be altered in some cases, like in margarine. Vegetable oils are hydrogenated—have hydrogens added to them—to make them more saturated and more solid, resulting in margarines.

It's important to understand the extent of saturation or unsaturation of foods because of the influence of saturation on the body's use of cholesterol. Cholesterol is a fat-like substance found naturally in the body. It is a normal ingredient in the blood and is found in every cell. Some of the cholesterol is made by the body and some comes from our food. Cholesterol is only found in foods of animal origin and is not present in plants (fruits, vegetables, grains, legumes, nuts, vegetable oils). The amount of cholesterol included in the diet is one factor that affects the level of cholesterol in the bloodstream. It is generally accepted that saturated fats tend to increase the cholesterol level in the blood, polyunsaturates decrease blood cholesterol, and monounsaturates have no significant affect either way. Therefore, when buying or eating food, go for the polyunsaturates (vegetable source) and ease up on the saturates (animal source).

Studies are showing that the presence of high blood cholesterol contributes to atherosclerosis disease in many people. Atherosclerosis is a progressive, deteriorating process where fatty substances flowing in the bloodstream are deposited on the inner walls of the arteries. In time the deposit enlarges to inhibit the flow of blood and it eventually may block the entire artery. This ends the supply of nutrients and oxygen to the particular tissue that this artery feeds, and the tissue dies. When an artery in the brain is blocked some of the brain tissue dies and the result is a stroke. When an artery in the heart itself, a coronary artery, becomes blocked, part of the heart tissue dies and becomes ineffective, it's a heart attack. Either can be fatal—or, at best, disabling. So consider cholesterol to be one item in a group of risk factors that lead to heart disease. This does not mean that everyone should radically change their diets for there are no guarantees, but rather use moderation in total fat consumption as well as prudently approaching the other risk factors, including blood pressure, smoking, obesity, heredity and low level of exercise.

Water-hydration

Water is a nutrient essential for life. It is as important as oxygen for breathing. You can live without food for days or even up to two weeks, but you can only last a few days without water.

About two-thirds of the body weight is water. Water serves as a building material, a solvent for all products of digestion, the medium of body fluids—secretions and excretions—a regulator of body temperature by means of evaporation through skin and lungs, a carrier of nutrients and waste products from one part of the body to another, an aid in digestion, and it is a necessary part in all chemical reactions of metabolism.

The right amount of water is maintained in the body by a part of the brain controlling thirst. When your body is running low in water, you feel thirsty—you are dehydrated. **Dehydration leads to fatigue and poor flying performance.** When there is too much water, it is excreted by the kidneys in urine. You cannot drink too much water, especially while flying.

Water losses need to be replaced in the body every day in generous amounts. Water usually is supplied by drinking, but there also is water in foods. There is no magic number of glasses of water that you should consume every day. Instead, let nature be your guide.

Vitamins and Minerals

In terms of quantity or mass, our foods consist mostly of protein, carbohydrates, fats and water. These substances are extremely important in building a healthy body but would be useless without certain other supplies—the vitamins and minerals. The vitamins and minerals are smaller in quantity and not as visible, but they are essential in building and maintaining a human body.

Vitamins are quite popular in the health scene today. Many people are aware of the importance of vitamins and know that they are essential for health and survival of all living things. There are controversies, however, as to what amount of each vitamin should be included in the diet. It is important that we get the right amounts because either too little *or* too much of a vitamin can cause serious illnesses. We use vitamins in extremely minute amounts, milligrams and micrograms, so even a seemingly small amount in excess can be toxic in certain vitamins. It is erroneous to assume with vitamins or any other drug chemical that "if a little of something is good, then a lot is better." But still, the per-capita consumption of vitamins is steadily increasing in the pill-popping United States.

Vitamins have dynamic functions in body processes, regulating many chemical reactions. They are essential for the release of energy from food, for normal growth of different tissues of the body, for controlling the body's use of food, and for proper functioning of nerves and muscles. They do *not* provide energy or build tissues. They have no calories.

About 14 major vitamins have been identified (there may be more) that are necessary for health. Recommended amounts have been established for ten of them. Each vitamin has a special function in the body and no other nutrient can take its place or do its job. So, once again, a variety of foods is important in order to get the variety of vitamins.

Vitamins can be categorized into two classes, depending on whether they are soluble in fat or soluble in water. The water-soluble viatmins—C, thiamin, niacin and riboflavin—are able to be mixed in water as a solution. They are *not* stored by the body. Excesses of the water soluble vitamins are excreted in the urine. When taken in large doses these vitamins may be creating very expensive urine! That's a waste.

The fat soluble vitamins—A, D, E and K—are stored by the body and are not flushed out in the urine. They are not soluble in water, so care must be taken with these because too much A, D, E or K can cause toxic amounts to build up in the body.

Are you getting enough vitamins? Should you be taking some vitamin supplements? Are you overdosing on any vitamins already? The answers to these questions are not simple. Obviously, it is impossible for you to know exactly what is taking place inside your own cells down to the microgram level. But a tremendous amount of research has been conducted to establish some guidelines for eating and some requirements for daily intake of vitamins. The investigations continue and modifications are made in the guidelines as more and more evidence is revealed. In the meantime you need to be wise about your eating practices. A pattern of three or more small, regular meals each day, of a well-chosen *variety* of foods, taken in *moderation* should provide you with adequate amounts of vitamins.

If you have some way of knowing that you are not getting all of the nutrients that you need, if you are not eating right, if you are skipping meals, if you are not getting an assortment of fruits, vegetables, meats, milk and grains, or if you are replacing too many real foods with junk foods, then you need a conservative multivitamin supplement—not necessarily a mega-vitamin. Again, use careful moderation.

There are certain physical signs and symptoms that indicate excesses or deficiencies of vitamin function. If you suspect any of these, have a checkup by a physician who is qualified to do the appropriate tests and prescribe a supplement for the specific condition. The condition usually is more complex than it seems, so seek advice. Self-diagnosis and self-treatment by altering your own vitamin intake can be dangerous, especially when tampering with one vitamin disproportionately to the others. It may upset the delicate balance between the different vitamins, and may even distract you from noticing a much more serious disease process going on in your body. For example, you wouldn't want to be consuming mega-doses of Vitamin D, believing that it will relieve your abdominal discomfort when what you really have is an ulcer, or a bacterial infection, or a tumor, or cancer, that is going unnoticed and untreated while you're busy with vitamin D. An additional problem with self-treatment is that you may really be eating the right amount of a particular vitamin, but something is wrong within the body so it is *not using* the vitamin even though it is available. This is an absorption problem, and increasing the quantity of the vitamin intake is futile. Seek medical advice.

Vitamins are indispensible and play a vital role in keeping us healthy by assisting in numerous processes of growth and development. They inhibit diseases such as scurvy, beri-beri, anemia, and rickets. Lately, the vitamin industry is profiting from many misleading claims made about the use of some vitamins by promising all sorts of miraculous rewards such as endless energy and physical endurance, a better sex life, instant relief from colds, guaranteed good health, slowing of the aging process, elimination of body odor, prevention of grey hair, etc. Vitamins do contribute to feeling great but be leary of exaggerations and single incidents that are not yet supported by scientific evidence. Also, be aware that as a result of frivolous, superficial advertising and a rather careless public attitude, vitamins have developed the connotation of being simple, harmless, colorful, candied "kidstuff." Actually vitamins are chemicals with very complex molecular structures and long chemical names. Eating excessive amounts of vitamins may have adverse side effects. Some of the symptoms of hypervitaminosis are; fatigue, weight loss, pains, skin changes, loss of appetite, changes in elimination, abdominal discomfort, insomnia, high blood pressure, headache, nausea, vomiting, etc. Massive doses of certain vitamins can cause death. So vitamins should be handled seriously and carefully like any drug.

About four to five percent of your total body weight is made up of minerals, another group of nutrients essential for living. They are natural elements that have important contributions to make to vital body functions. About 15 are known to be required and daily recommended allowances have been established for six of them. Like the vitamins, minerals do not provide calories, so they do not supply energy. They are not broken down in the body but are absorbed from the digestive track in the same form as they occur in the foods. Minerals are not "used up" by the body, but enter, carry out their specific function, and are excreted. This is why minerals must be replaced regularly by daily eating a good, balanced, varied diet. (Iron is the exception. It is stored and reused.) If you are not eating adequate meals, consider taking a moderate daily supplement. The following are some highlights of the most prominent minerals.

Calcium is the most abundant mineral in the body—about two-to-three pounds' worth. Almost all of it is concentrated in the bones and teeth, giving them strength and rigidity. The small amount of calcium in the rest of the body tissues and fluids aids in the clotting of the blood, the contraction of muscles, transmission of nerve impulses, heart functions, regulation of fluids and activation of enzymes. Calcium deficiency results in rickets (in children) and osteoporosis, the softening of the bones. Calcium is found especially in milk and cheeses.

Phosphorus also is a main ingredient along with calcium for building bones and teeth. It also helps regulate energy within the body cells. It is easily obtained; good sources are meat, poultry, fish, eggs and whole-grain foods.

Iodine is vital to the normal function of the thyroid gland, which controls metabolism. It is required in extremely small amounts but getting too little can cause goiter, a swelling of the thyroid gland in the neck. People who live inland where the soil contains little iodine sometimes fail to get adequate amounts. Iodized table salt and seafoods are good sources of iodine.

Iron is needed in small but important amounts. It combines with protein to make hemoglobin, the red substance of blood that carries oxygen to the cells and carbon dioxide to the lungs to be exhaled. Too little iron in the diet or chronic blood loss can cause iron deficiency anemia. Liver is an excellent source of iron. Other sources are organ meats, shellfish, lean meats, egg yolks, dark green leafy vegetables, dried fruit, molasses and whole-grain cereals.

Other minerals include: chlorine, cobalt, copper, fluorine, magnesium, potassium, manganese, sodium, sulfur, zinc, chromium, selenium and molybdenum.

THE CHECKLIST

Checklists, checklists, checklists . . . As a pilot you are more than familiar with the idea of using checklists. The checklist is a list of things to do in a certain order. It serves as a tool in accomplishing a specific task, whether that be a preflight or an emergency procedure. The purpose of each checklist is to make the task easier, faster, safer and more accurate. It insures that no items are missed. Following a systematic, progressive checklist simplifies the job for the pilot, saves valuable time in situations where seconds count and limits the possibility of human error.

In a similar fashion, when it comes to eating properly, there are special checklists, too. By faithfully following these eating checklists you can be assured that you are getting all of the nutrients that you need each day. They are quite accurate, very simple to use and virtually effortless.

Why bother? Well, considering the three basic nutrients—protein, carbohydrates and fat—plus all of the different vitamins, and adding all of the minerals, you've got about 40 to 50 total nutrients to keep track of. If you had nothing better to do, you could befriend a computer and spend all of your waking hours in scientific research in an attempt to determine by yourself your individual nutrient needs, and then try to calculate exactly how many micrograms of this 'n that should actually go down the hatch. But, as a pilot who would rather spend your time flying, you're in luck: Nutrition scientists have done the hard part already. As a result of years of research and surveys they have provided us with information such as in the *Nutritive Value of American Foods, Handbook #456,* published by the U.S.D.A. On a smaller scale this information has been reduced to lists of recommended daily allowances of each nutrient for special ages and energy needs. These lists are periodically reviewed and revised to incorporate new findings. They are intended to be recommendations for all healthy people; the amounts that are given in the "recommended daily allowances" (RDA) are generous enough to accommodate the individual variations among the normal population living in the United States who are under normal amounts of environmental stress. They serve as a guide for planning food intake.

The knowledge of the nutrient needs of people and the nutritive content of our foods has been translated from technical language into an easily understood food guide for everyday use. This daily food checklist arranges foods into four groups according to content, because certain types of food have common nutrients occurring in approximately the same quantity. Each food usually contains more than one type of nutrient, but no single food supplies all 40 to 50 nutrients. So it is important to eat a *variety* of foods in *moderation*. Based on the amounts of each nutrient needed daily for proper growth, maintenance and repair, scientists were able to recommend the amount of foods to eat in terms of number of servings from each of four general food groups. How much more convenient could this be? All you have to know is this easy checklist.

      Meat Group - 2 servings per day
      Milk Group - 2
      Fruit/Veg. - 4
      Grains - 4

If this idea looks vaguely familiar, that's because you may remember it from grade school. In case you think it is too simple or too old-fashioned, remember that this is not just a fleeting fad or a temporary theory. It was not contrived by scientific minds, but rather, it is a recognizable pattern that is part of creation. Thank heaven we are not limited to only one kind of food. In contrast, you can choose from an endless assortment to suit personal taste, family budget, caloric need, stage of life, and need for weight control. The food-group pattern for a healthy diet is the same as it has been for many years, but we have learned better how to "alter to fit" for individual needs within the guidelines.

If this is still too much to ask you to understand, at least try to keep in mind two very important concepts as you plan your meals . . . VARIATION . . . and MODERATION!

Thermodynamics for Aerodynamics

Nutrition, as well as aeronautics, engineering, chemistry, physics, ecology and all disciplines, is subject to laws of nature—laws that exist as an intrinsic part of creation and are not contrived by any of our own human machinations. They are inescapable.

You are currently flying an incredible piece of equipment but even that enormous machine has limitations. Powerful as it is, it still must submit to the laws of nature. Each aircraft has its own particular maximum take-off weight and maximum landing weight, for instance. These numerical values impose the upper limit of safety for the particular aerodynamics of that structure. It would be dangerous to ignore such limitations and attempt to operate the aircraft beyond its capabilities; even the guy who loves to push the envelope knows he can't put a max-grossed 747 into a vertical climb.

So what about you, the pilot of the aircraft? Consider your limits governed by the laws of nature. Each cell of your body is far more intricate than the aircraft. You are a veritable container of infinitely complex chemical reactions that miraculously continue in spite of your abuse. Your heart labors unceasingly to sustain your life. What are its limits? When you "took-off" this morning to start your day were you at your ideal weight or were you carrying 10 or 20 pounds of extra baggage? Were you maintaining an airworthy anatomy? Are you putting undue stress on your heart muscle? Like with your aircraft, if you tax your heart beyond its natural limits, something will give.

When an airplane is overgross with fuel beyond the maximum landing weight, there are two alternatives: burn it or dump it. You can continue in flight and burn fuel at the normal rates of consumption. A faster method is to dump fuel—simply drop the excess from the plane. When over gross physically, wouldn't it be wonderful to be able to simply dump the excess "baggage" from your body? It would be great if the flab would just melt off. Fortunately and unfortunately, the human body doesn't work that way. The body is actually a more efficient machine than the aircraft. As a means of self-preservation, the body clutches any excess food fuel, stores it as fat, and saves it for a possible future time when fuel may be scarce—planning ahead for hard times. But in our culture today our "storehouses" are full to overflowing and we experience few hard times. No dumping is possible. The method of choice is to burn the extra fat and lighten the load for the overworked heart.

Each of us is a self-contained system of matter and energy, and like every other organism we are subject to some inescapable laws of nature governing development, growth and change. Our physical equilibrium, or health, depends on these unchanging natural laws for the complex chemical reactions of matter and the conservation of energy (heat) within the system, the body. We cannot defy the laws of chemodynamics and thermodynamics which rule the human machine. But we can use these scientific properties to our advantage in maintaining health.

Airworthy Anatomy

To maintain good health and an ideal weight you need to know your system and the laws that govern it. Don't be swayed by pushers of magical foods and hocus-pocus diets which claim to circumvent the natural processes and promise immediate results. They usually amount to an expense to your health and your pocket. You need to know the principles of matter and energy as they relate to the functions of eating and exercise as a basis for good health. There is very little value to the temporary, two-week diet. Instead, develop a sensible eating style *for life*.

The human machine is able to unlock usable energy from its fuel, food. It has the capability of chemically breaking down the three foodstuffs, protein, carbohydrates and fats (or amino acids, simple sugars and fatty acids, respectively) to create "free energy". Whenever chemical bonds are broken, energy is released. Using an amazing bodily process, this free energy is not lost as heat but instead it is carefully transferred to a specialized molecule called ATP. In this new form, the energy can be stored in the cells of the body to be used later at the precise time of need, whether it be for a heartbeat, a game of racquetball or ruddering an aircraft. The more vigorous the activity, the more ATP's will give up their energy.

Energy from food is measured in units called calories (technically kilocalories but shortened in the U.S.). All foods supply calories, but some supply many more than others. Calories are not nutrients; rather they are a means of expressing the amount of potential energy for bodily use that can be released from the nutrients. (Getting really scientific, a calorie is the amount of heat needed to raise the temperature of one pint of water by four degrees Fahrenheit.)

The daily amount of energy you need, in terms of calories, depends mostly on your particular body size and your level of physical activity—or inactivity. Some other influencing factors are your age, sex and stage of growth. At rest your body requires about one calorie per minute just to work at staying alive by maintaining the minimum functions. It's like idling your engine. The motor is running but you're not going anywhere. Some people exist this way—just barely "on" while always avoiding any extra exertion. The problem is that they may eat as much as others who *are* active.

Eating fats, carbohydrates and proteins supplies the raw materials for growth and energy production when you need it. But eating an overabundance of them doesn't make you more "energetic." In fact, eating more than you need causes storage of these materials in the form of adipose tissue. In plain terms the excess makes you fat and sluggish, not more active.

Danger! Excess calories may be hazardous to your health! Whether fats, proteins, or carbohydrates, a calorie . . . is a calorie . . . is a calorie, no matter where it came from and —get this—3,500 unused calories make 1 pound of body fat.

The accumulation of the 3,500 unburned calories may be sudden, as during holiday seasons when people excuse themselves from restraints, or it may be almost imperceptible—a few calories here and a few more calories there and soon a pound sneaks up on you. Consider this situation: every day for one year you ate 100 calories in excess of what you need—just 100 calories each day beyond the point where you should have stopped. It may be in the form of a nutritious food, or, sad to say, it may have been of the junk variety. It may have looked like this:

	100 calories more
1st day — a medium apple	than what you needed
2nd day — a cookie	"
3rd day — 8 potato chips	"
4th day — ⅔ cup milk	"
5th day — 1 Tbs. butter	"
6th day — 1 slice of lunchmeat	"
(getting the idea?)	
363rd day — 1 orange	"
364th day — 1 Tbs. salad dressing	"
365th day — 1 Tbs. cream in your coffee	"

The list looks pretty harmless, doesn't it. And a lot of the items are even good for you. *But,* 100 extra calories each day, whether from a nutritious apple or a junky cookie, for one year gives you 10 pounds of excess fat. *10 Pounds!* In one year! Gasp!

You can easily see that if this process is allowed to continue obesity develops. Calories *do* count! Just try counting yours and you will see. You can't change the laws of nature or escape them. But you can understand them and then use them to your benefit instead of being destroyed by them. Try putting the process in reverse and *lose* 10 pounds instead! When the number of calories that you eat is equal to the number of calories that you use, your weight will remain stable because a balance is achieved. When calories eaten exceed calories used, you will **gain** weight. When calories eaten are fewer than calories used, you will **lose** weight.

There are no magic foods or diets that flush fat out of the body. NONE. Weight gain, loss, or stability is a matter of simple arithmetic addition and subtraction. The way to lose weight is to burn more calories than you eat or eat less than you burn. Create a calorie deficit. The best way is to eat less and exercise more!

Any eating/activity pattern (I avoid using the word "diet" because it implies something *temporary*) that creates a deficit in calories will cause you to lose weight. But since our goal is to stay slim *and* healthy, not merely slim, be sure that the foods that you do eat are the nutritious ones. While you are counting calories you might as well throw out the foods that are purely empty calories, such as soda pop and sweets. They are of no value to you. Emphasize foods that are packed with good things, vitamins and minerals. They are a better investment.

Most people are at their ideal weight sometime between the age of 20 and 25. After that, fewer and fewer calories are needed to keep the ideal weight, but people usually continue to eat the same amounts anyway just out of habit. That's appetite, not hunger. There is a difference. Also, in later years they become less physically active, which further contributes pounds.

Prevention is the name of the game when it comes to your health. By periodically and routinely checking your bodily "guages" and "indicators" for potential health risks, you may save your life and maybe the lives of those on board. A thorough "physical pre-flight" can identify a possible problem in its early stages, in time for you to reduce the risk and thereby increase your years of good health and life expectancy. You have some built-in early warning systems if you will just stop and notice them.

Develop a risk-factor consciousness for an effective physical pre-flight. Risk factors are those characteristics of your medical history, your family history, and your medical status that are linked with high rates of premature death and disability from certain diseases. Risk is a statistical expression of probability of a greater likelihood of disease, your personal early warning system. The pertinent risk factors are such things as a high level of blood cholesterol, smoking, high blood pressure, diabetes, overweight, inappropriate diet, stress, age, sex, lack of exercise, an abnormal electrocardiogram, and heredity.

As you are inspecting your human machine in your physical pre-flight, do you find any indications of overgross? You don't have to look very hard; its usually pretty obvious. Remember that calories *do* count, and the two key points to good eating—moderation and variation.

The advantages of being at your best weight are more than worth the effort involved in taking off the rolls around the middle. Besides looking your best, it gives you wonderful fringe benefits:
1. Reduces risk of heart attack
2. Reduces risk of stroke
3. Helps to prevent or delay diabetes
4. Lowers blood pressure
5. Lowers blood fat and buildup of athersclerosis

In terms of the future, some of your risk factors can be modified or even removed. In so doing, you can positively change your health and maybe increase your overall life expectancy. You may not be able to do much about your sex, heredity and your age, but you can work on the other risk factors (blood pressure, smoking, diet, weight, exercise, and stress) to give you more years of health, and maybe more years. There still are no guarantees, but reducing your risks will give you the best chance of escaping a heart attack in your prime, productive years.

IN BRIEF

Incorporating healthy eating habits and proper physical activity into your routine lifestyle can greatly enhance and probably extend your productive years. An attitude of preventive health maintenance is far better than blindly waiting for some eventual mishap to jolt you into a panic-stricken awareness of your need for change.

Whether shopping for groceries, preparing a meal, eating at home, enjoying a dinner party, sneaking a snack, ordering in a restaurant, consuming a crew meal, pot-lucking at a picnic, or raiding the refrigerator, the same philosophy in making food choices should prevail in all situations. It should be a subconscious, automatic decision to make the best possible food choice in each case. Use wisdom in developing a prudent eating style, and not the ups-and-downs of temporary flings and binges. Here are some helps:

- Eat a wide *variety* of foods from each of the four food groups.
- Eat *moderate* amounts. Overeating is hazardous to your health.
- Emphasize foods in their original state—fresh fruit, fresh vegetables, whole grains.
- De-emphasize animal products—beef, pork, butter, eggs—and heavily processed foods.
- Beware of table salt and white sugar. Also watch out for sodium and sugars hidden in processed foods.
- Elminiate the "unfoods" with the empty calories like pop, candy, sweets.
- Read nutrition labels for calorie content and nutrient breakdown. Ingredient lists are usually arranged in order of decreasing amounts. If a sugar, sodium, nitrites, or other villains are listed early in the list, select a different item.
- Eat slowly. Take more time to enjoy the flavor and texture of each different food. Try new foods.

If you are trying to lose weight you still need to eat right as discussed above, but in addition, you need to burn more calories than you eat, or eat less than you burn. Shedding the flab is possible, but there is no immediate, safe, magical way. Avoid the extremes of fad reducing diets and gimmicks. They may appear to be effective temporarily, but in the long run can be harmful to your health. A slow, careful change in your long-range eating style is best. A wide variety of

foods eaten in MODERATION is your best bet. Remember that 3,500 calories makes one pound, so cut back on calories at meals and snacks. Calories *do* count! Create a calorie deficit and you will lose weight. Here are some more helps:
- Since calories count, count 'em! Try keeping a food diary for several days listing foods eaten, portion sizes, and number of calories. It will be an "eye-opener." You will be able to identify problem foods in your personal diet and eliminate them. It's not as boring as it sounds. Many pilots have done it.
- Snacks, beverages and "tastes" have calories too!
- Diet pills do not work, the diet does. In addition, these pills can raise your blood pressure to unacceptable levels.
- Limit fats, refined sugar and alcoholic beverages.
- Work with someone who has the same goals. It's amazing how much more diligent we are when held accountable to someone else.
- Prepare your plate with care. Don't surround yourself with bowls of food at the table which "tease" you into taking seconds. You don't even have to eat everything on your plate.
- EXERCISE! Physical activity is a great help. It burns calories and curbs the appetite.
- Put a copy of your medical certificate on your refrigerator door as a reminder of how important your health is.

8

An Exercise Program for Pilots

A 35-year-old airline pilot was noted to have a "variation" in his EKG, and since it was the first one submitted to the FAA, he was asked by the FAA for more evaluation. The pilot was out of shape, had a high resting pulse rate, and was a heavy coffee drinker. His obviously poor condition was "cured" by an exercise program, and he stopped drinking excessive coffee. His EKG returned to normal. However, the additional evaluation turned out to be OK, eventhough it also had to be reported to the FAA instead of being kept confidential.

THE 1970s SAW an increased interest by Americans in physical fitness and general "wellness." No longer was the lone jogger someone to stare at. This awareness of "wellness" was not a passing fad: As more people became involved and realized the benefits, others began to take notice and begin their own exercise programs. Such programs have stood the test of time, and in the majority of cases, have withstood comments from critics. The concept of health maintenance is alive and well.

However, if such programs are so beneficial, why is it that more people are not participating? If an exercise program truly prolongs life and maintains one's good health and sense of well-being, why are not all professional pilots participating in some sort of exercise program? Nobody said it was easy to maintain your health, and certainly beginning and continuing an exercise program is not a simple task. But with a career at stake, why the apathy?

Let's begin by defining why exercise is important both physiologically and psychologically. Unlike more mechanical machines, the human machine performs better, more efficiently and longer if it is worked under controlled conditions. This leads to a "quality of health" that all of us envy. What then are the special qualities found after participating in an active exercise program?

First, there is an improved efficiency of our lungs. We are better able to use the air (oxygen) that we inhale, and better at exhaling the impurities and carbon dioxide. Those who exercise realize that they no longer have to huff and puff for usual, mildly strenuous activities such as going up and down stairs. Their capacity for work has increased and the necessity to breath harder when working has decreased. They finally can keep up with their children without having to slow down and blame it all on age.

Equally important is the improvement of heart *muscle.* This heart muscle is like other muscles in the body that weaken and become flabby without strenuous use. Granted, the heart is pumping all the time, but only in a mild way, especially if we lead a sedentary life. Just as calisthenics and weight lifting increase the mass of those muscles used during those exercises, the only way we can provide the same sort of exercise to the heart muscle is to make it work harder over a prolonged period. Those who participate in an exercise program notice that they can tolerate the stress of hard work and prolonged exercise with much greater ease without a pounding heart and racing pulse. They also notice that the resting pulse is lower than it used to be. That is, instead of being at 88 in a resting situation, it is now in the 60s. Obviously, that lower pulse rate is an indication that the heart muscle is far more efficient than it used to be, and needs to beat less frequently; it has far more efficient hydraulic pressure with each beat.

An unexpected, but pleasant, spin-off of a physical-conditioning program is a general feeling of well-being. The entire body feels better, fatiques less easily, and one has a general attitude of having more energy. The body is also far more resistant to diseases and other complications that result from the abuses to which we subject it in our daily life.

Contrary to popular opinion, an exercise program is not the sole method for weight loss. In other words, you cannot go out and run a mile and then come back and gorge yourself with all the food that you know you shouldn't be eating and expect to lose weight. Remember, one pound of fat is equal to about 3,500 calories. You can either walk, run or jog *one* mile, but you will use only 100 calories. In order to burn off the pound of fat you have stored and accumulated by overeating, you would have to run 35 miles! That is a pretty high price to pay for your over-indulgence. Exercise does use up calories, though, and certainly over time it is a great companion to a weight-reduction program. In other words, you usually can't lose weight efficiently without adopting some sort of exercise program *along with your diet.* For example, if you were to walk an extra mile a day, that's 100 calories burned. If you also eat 100 calories less a day, that's a total of 200 calories, and over a month's period, that's about 6,000 calories, or about two pounds of weight loss. It requires discipline, but the combination is more rewarding and lasting if you are willing to wait for the results.

So how can you tell if you are improving your physical condition from a good program? What are the tangible and objective results that you can see? Probably the most important is your pulse rate. We should all be familiar with our *resting* pulse rate. (It should be no more than 75 and ideally in the low 60s.) With moderate exercise, your pulse shouldn't go much above 150, and it should return to normal or slightly above resting rate after a minimal amount of rest (10 to 20 minutes). This is an indication that the heart is working efficiently, and its *muscle* is in good physical condition. Get in the habit of frequently checking your pulse.

Your blood pressure, if elevated, will also begin to come down, but not as noticeably as your pulse rate. You might also notice an increased ability to tolerate the stresses of life, whether they be psychological or physical, far more efficiently. Although somewhat subjective in definition, you will notice that you will have more energy and will be able to partake more in life's everyday enjoyments, rather than calling it quits after returning home from a long trip.

You will feel good and you will look good. People will begin to notice that you are a different person, and you will begin to realize that the way you used to feel is not a good feeling after all, certainly not worth the sacrifice necessary to over-indulge in food, cigarettes, alcohol. etc. Exercise is the key to an over-all physical conditioning program. As a result, your personal needs for a good quality of life will not *require* the social abuses in which Americans indulge.

You will find yourself suffering from fewer colds and flus, and if you do have an illness you will bounce back much quicker. Obviously, no one can guarantee total absence of illness, but certainly you can return to flying much sooner than somebody whose sedentary life has resulted in a generalized poor physical condition.

If there are so many good points about exercise, let's examine for a moment why so many of us do not participate in an exercise program. What is it that keeps you from doing something that would keep you certified and healthy? The biggest problem is pure laziness, which unfortunately is a result of not exercising. Therefore, it is a vicious circle. You just can't seem to get started. In addition, we expect immediate results. Once we are turned on to an exercise program, if we don't see these results in a few days, we become discouraged and slip back into our old habits. As a pilot, you are used to seeing your efforts reach fruition within a matter of minutes or hours, and you can see the results of your work at the end of the day. This certainly is not true in an exercise program. Therefore, we rationalize and find excuses for not beginning an exercise program. The excuses include its being "too boring" and "I never have enough time," "it's too lonely," "I don't know where to exercise," "I would rather spend the time with my family," etc. You and I have heard all of these before, and I am sure that each of you have also expressed them. Until you have actually experienced the feelings of being in good physical condition, an exercise program won't likely become a top priority—you'll always have other things to do. Interestingly, those who do find time to exercise tend to be *more* efficient in the use of their over-all time and accomplish far more than those who do not.

Unfortunately, one of the greatest incentives to begin an exercise program is when the AME tells a pilot that, because of his general poor physical fitness, his blood pressure is too high and he is grounded until he can get it lowered. One can imagine the efforts that a pilot now will make to achieve a necessary exercise program. Fortunately, in these cases the pilot will realize what he has been missing and will continue to participate in this physical conditioning since he does not want to feel the way he used to. He will become proud of the way he looks and the fact that he is able to maintain his endurance under conditions which he wasn't able to tolerate in the past.

But being grounded is a poor way to get your attention. A better way is to commit yourself to another person, be it your spouse, a friend or someone else who has the same problems in getting started and continuing. You must, however, accept the fact that you need an exercise program before you can subject yourself to the eventual problems you will face in starting and continuing the program. It's a commitment. Until you begin to notice the good results and benefits, the job will be tough. Being a pilot—with irregular hours, staying overnight in various locations, and actually being too fatigued to participate in a program because of a long trip—does create a realistic and actual deterrent to developing a good program. However, once you have seriously defined the need, you can begin to look into the possibilities. I am sure you will be pleasantly surprised to find a number of people faced with the same complications who have been able to resolve the difficulties and are now following a commendable physical conditioning program. These are the people you should talk with. Allow them to share their methods and ways of overcoming the deterrents. Once you have faced the issue of needing to start a program, and—I hope—have found someone to share the program with, you must choose a type of exercise and schedule it so it will be productive for you. You probably will have to develop two programs; one that you can practice at home and one you can do on trips.

Many people think that an exercise program is limited to jogging. Jogging turns some people off, and if that's your feeling, then jogging is not what you should be doing. There are many alternatives, and certainly jogging is not the only answer. There are many excellent books that address the issue of an exercise program, and they do not advocate jogging as the sole source for the most efficient results. Admittedly, jogging is one of the most efficient, but it does take a commitment of time and sacrifice of other activities. Some of the better books include *The New Aerobics* by Kenneth H. Cooper, M.D., and a pamphlet entitled "Beyond Diet: Exercise your Way to Fitness and Heart Health" by Lenore R. Zohman, M.D., which usually can be found at your local American Heart Association office.

All the respected and accepted books on exercise programs basically have one goal in mind, and that is what we will discuss now. One word of caution: Even a little exercise is better than nothing, provided that it is not the type where you exert yourself beyond your capacities during a short period once a week. It is better to commit yourself to a few minutes a day and then build up to a more complete program rather than try to make up for lost time on the weekends. The "weekend athlete" is a prime target for sudden medical disorders, not only heart attacks, but sprained ankles, sore backs, etc., all of which prevent the pursuit of future programs. It is better to start out slowly and work up gradually. The other extreme is someone who gets so turned on by an exercise program that he becomes extremely competitive and starts running seven, eight or even nine miles a day, playing aggressive handball, etc. to the point where he is risking injury. Such an injury could limit his exercise so severely that he returns to his old ways.

The "secret" to a any good exercise program is simply this: After a ten-minute warm-up of stretching, walking, calisthenics, walking in place, or so on, progress into a period of exercise that raises your pulse to the target rate specific for your age and keep it there for about 20 minutes. Then gradually cool down for another 10 minutes by either slowing the activities or going back to the calisthenics, slow walking, etc. At no time should you jump into vigorous exercise and then suddenly stop and go about your usual business. A warm-up, cool-down and stretching program is essential. Forty-to-60 minutes, two-to-three times a week, certainly is not much of a sacrifice of time, but it is amazing how often we can rationalize allegedly better uses for those few moments. Another part of this "secret" is that you should not allow more than two or three days to elapse between your exercise.

Pulse is an indicator of how you are doing. Keep a record of your pulse. Know what your resting pulse is, how long it takes you to get up to your target rate, and how long it takes you to get down to your resting pulse after your exercise. Techniques for determining what these rates should be and how they can be improved are more fully explained in the books mentioned previously.

An incentive you might use is to keep a chart with resting, exercising and cool-down pulses. Post them where everybody can see it; that way you can't cheat. You might put a copy of your medical certificate right on top of this graph to remind you of why you're going to the trouble. Doing this next to a diet and weight chart also is a strong motivator. This is even better if you can begin to compete with a member of your family or a friend so you can keep track of each other's progress and give support to continue.

The type of exercise best for you is probably the hardest thing to determine. Again, books very nicely explain the alternatives and how they relate to each other in terms of output and efficiency. In addition to jogging, running and walking, don't forget about jumping rope, small mini-trampolines that can be used in the house, stationary bikes and treadmills, and of course competitive sports. Many of those you can do at home, but they're somewhat more difficult for you to pursue when you are on a trip. If you check into a motel where you can either go swimming or go up and down several flights of stairs, jump rope or just go for a long walk, you've found an ideal place to stay. Certainly with your health and career at stake, it would behoove you to find places where your exercise program can be followed. It is my understanding that many hotels and motels are providing access to exercise facilities for guests.

To review: I recommend reading a few books that will give you alternative ways to achieve the goal of increasing your pulse over a gradual period of time, keeping it there for a minimum of 20 minutes, and then a cool-down period. Even if you are not sure how you are going to like it, at least go out and buy the jump rope or jogging shoes or even the mini-trampoline. Commit yourself to at least three or four weeks before you decide that you don't want or can't pursue the program. Talk with others. Find out how they resolve their hangups. Most important of all, do something, share it with somebody else, and keep a record.

9

Habits and Abuses that Affect Your Certification, and Miscellaneous Medical Topics

THE FOLLOWING SUBJECTS are common, and I have mentioned them all throughout this book. Each can be controlled by self-commitment and self-control. We all can identify with these habits, we see them in ourselves and in our flying comrades, habits which vary in each individual from abstinance to partaking of all.

As a professional pilot, you picked a career which means that in addition to applying love of flying, you must maintain your health. Each one of these subjects can affect that vital medical certificate. Those who combined these factors are asking for an even more probable disappointing future. I discuss them not to bring up something you weren't aware of, but to keep you conscious of their effects on your health and ultimately your flying career. Perhaps when you reach for a cigarette or that extra cup of coffee or that last, "one for the road," you'll think of some of the comments made in this book.

SMOKING

Everyone knows that smoking is bad. Everyone knows that smoking is a major risk factor in developing heart disease and pulmonary complications. Nobody has been able to justify why he or she smokes other than habit brought on initially by enjoyment. Yet smoking continues to be the sole source of nicotine, a very strong stimulant to the heart and blood vessels; a major cause of malignancies, and a source of carbon monoxide which adds to your already hypoxic condition while flying. If you wish to have a choice of which disease you can acquire, pick cancer because of its finality. Emphysema is a horrible way to live because it is very difficult to breath under even the most minimal of exertions. Bronchitis is a continuing and progressive source of infection. As we had stated earlier, significant coronary artery disease is a mandatory disqualification. With emphysema, chronic bronchitis or coronary artery disease, you have to live with it for an indefinite time. At least with cancer, your future is more fully defined.

The carbon monoxide of a burning cigarette is a major factor leading to increased hypoxia, decreased night vision, and more noticeable fatigability, especially after a trip. Often those who smoke also consume vast amounts of caffeine, which means that the "let down" from this over-stimulated state (after the trip) is a situation that prevents you from relaxing as you should.

Equally important is the insult to those who do not like or cannot tolerate smoke in the cockpit. This, plus dry air, is one of the most common complaints pilots have about their flying buddies. Not only are you insulting your colleagues, you are subjecting them to the same medical abuses that *you* have chosen, made worse in that confined, dry environment.

Very few smokers don't want to stop. A few have succeeded, most have at least cut down (which is *very* important—cutting down *improves* your risks), but there are those who continue to be heavy smokers in spite of the facts. It seems apparent to me, as a doctor, that I cannot scare the smoker; he is already aware of the harm it is doing. I suggest to those who want to quit that they must first truly want to; and if they don't, they might as well not even try. Their frustrations will be taken out not only on themselves, but on those around them. As with other bad habits, controlling your smoking cannot always be resolved alone. You should have someone with whom to do it. If you are willing to commit yourself to somebody else and establish your priorities with another person, they can be supportive and lend you guidance during the more tempting moments. Many support groups and many techniques have been tried, and they may be worthwhile if they get the job done. But if you can't do it for yourself, do it at least for those who depend upon you and care about you. It is difficult enough to put up with the stench of smoke on your breath and in your clothes. The sight of cigarettes, the tobacco and ash scattered throughout your clothes, and the risk that you are facing is hard enough to justify. But as a professional pilot, denying yourself and your family a career simply because you like your cigarettes is a perfect example of someone who has their priorities all turned around.

CAFFEINE

Coffee and tea are almost a part of our social lifestyle and certainly a part of the "after takeoff check list." The caffeine found in coffee, tea, most cola products and some chocolates, however, is more than the simple stimulant to get us going in the morning. To some this caffeine is a very strong stimulant to the heart muscle. In addition, it affects our minds in the sense that it makes them over-sensitive, anxious and in some cases neurotic. I have known cases of pilots who have been grounded because of an abnormality in their EKG that was purely a result of too much **caffeine.** They had some extra pulses (PVC's) and other rhythm problems directly related to this over-stimulation. Caffeine also acts as a diuretic. That is, it promotes the excretion of urine. For example, you can drink one cup of coffee and urinate three cups of water. In an already desert-dry flight deck, this easily leads to dehydration and fatigue. Caffeine can be very troublesome to some stomachs. While it may not necessarily cause ulcers, it is an overstimulant to the acid secretions. Some decaffeinated coffee is equally irritating.

The problem with caffeine is not the drug itself, but the amount that many of us take in purely *habit* form. You don't normally need that second cup of coffee, especially when you are flying or working. It becomes more of a habit, something to do with our hands, and we could just as easily drink coffee-flavored hot water. Especially while flying, the over-stimulation of caffeine in addition to the hydrating effect leads to an over-tense state and fatigue, not only during the trip but especially afterwards. It prevents you from resting comfortably and relaxing. Therefore, the withdrawal effects after a trip are equally disabling.

Controlling your caffeine intake is no different than controlling any other habit. You must first identify what you are doing, how much caffeine you are taking, and then find a substitute. In most cases, the first cup of coffee at the beginning of the trip is perfectly acceptable. After that, however, find substitutes, such as juices, highly diluted decaffeinated coffee, non-cola beverages, etc. Certainly make a habit of drinking several cups of water between those other beverages. An important thing to keep in mind is that every time you are offered a cup of coffee, ask for something else, even if it's just a glass of water. I think you will find the results after the trip most satisfying.

ALCOHOL

One does not have to be an alcoholic to suffer the effects of even small amounts of alcohol in our system. This is especially true if we mean to keep our minds and bodies alert even 12 to 24 hours after taking in the alcohol. Most of us who drink alcoholic beverages do so because of the flavor and euphoric feeling that it gives us. But, in addition, it is a strong stimulant to the heart muscle and to the rest of the mind in the sense that it makes us more excitable and makes the heart work harder. This is why you feel the heart pumping harder the day after a good party. The problem is that if one were to plot the time of the euphoria from one highball, that effect lasts much **less** than the effects of the stimulant. Therefore, as we *maintain* our euphoric atti-

Habits and Abuses

tude with two or three or more drinks, we are actually cumulatively adding on to the **stimulant** curve. As a result, the euphoria aspect leaves in a matter of hours, but the stimulant effect will be around for 12 to 24 hours. In addition, it prevents us from getting our REM sleep (the sleep necessary for a completely rested body). Alcohol seems to have the same effect as barbituates. That is, it does not allow us to achieve a **beneficial** sleep. We may virtually pass out after a party, but we have not really been rested by the next morning. Again, this is the reason why we are so tired the morning after the night before.

In addition, alcohol acts as a diuretic, causing dehydration. However, it is not simply a matter of replacing water to recover. In fact, part of the "hangover" effect is the fluid volume within our bodies (since the diuretic effect of alcohol lasts for only a short period of time) which increases and then prevents us from losing more fluids. The thirst brought about by the alcohol replacing water in our **cells** adds even more fluids to our bodies. This added fluid, in addition to the blood vessel expansion, especially in our heads, leads to our miserable headaches.

We all know that as we drink more over the years, we can tolerate more; and therefore how alcohol affects us will depend greatly upon the conditions under which we are drinking. The consequences of alcohol can affect us not just eight hours, **but up to two days later** — just from the withdrawal effects, from the stimulative effects, and from the fatigue that results. The effect of alcohol on the stomach has led many an ulcer to bleed. The problem, of course, also remains that those who drink a lot often smoke a lot, and this combination can be devastating. Those who think drinking a lot of coffee the following morning will help are wrong. What they end up doing is compounding the already over-stimulated effects on the heart. The next time you experience the "morning after the night before," consider what you are feeling — the pounding heart, the headache, the dehydration, the fatigue. It often is much longer than 12 hours before you can return to normal. This can't be changed with extra coffee and all the other magic remedies. Consider how the leftover effects of alcohol and coffee, plus your already abusive habits while you are flying, will affect your performance and your future FAA exam. Reread FAR 91.11. It addresses not only the drinking of alcohol, but the effects of drinking. These **effects** are not limited to being drunk, but also relate to fatigue, hangover, etc.

OVER-THE-COUNTER MEDICATIONS

In essence, there is no such thing as a medicine that is safe at usual flying cabin altitude. In fact, it is illegal. Remember FAR 91.11 (a)(3) which states no medicines interfering with flying are legal.

Your response to any medication, whether it is prescribed or over-the-counter, may be different at 5,000 feet than at sea level. Many medications are sold over-the-counter for our own self-diagnosis and treatment, but they basically are pain pills that include only aspirin and Tylenol-like products, antihistamines and stimulants. For example, when reading the labels, most of those which end in -amine or -ine, such as chlorpheniramine, phenylpropanolamine, or ephedrine and phenylphrine, are dangerous while flying. All of these may cause serious problems, not only because the side-effects of the medicine are dangerous, but the *reason* you are taking the medication may also be dangerous to you while you are flying. Trying to overcome the symptoms of a cold (which in itself should ground you temporarily) by taking some antihistamines (which will make you drowsy) is an example of those small, insidious problems that snowball into major problems. If there is any doubt, you should ground yourself. You are not qualified to play doctor and treat yourself, especially as a pilot. Get into the habit of reading labels on some of these over-the-counter medications and see what it really is that you are taking. You will be surprised to find how many times they combine caffeine, antihistamines and stimulants, in addition to alcohol and aspirin, to do the job advertised. By diagnosing yourself, then treating yourself for a problem that you probably shouldn't be flying with anyway, you are only compounding the problems and adding burdens to your flying colleagues.

FATIGUE

Fatigue is something that we all experience, but to a pilot, it is not just the fatigue from overwork and long hours. It is a common complaint that although you are "guaranteed" so many hours of "crew rest," trying to get a good night's sleep in a strange bed, in a different town, at odd hours is persistently difficult, at best. There is no easy solution, other than avoiding those factors which make it more difficult to sleep. The various techniques of relaxation therapy (TM, biofeedback, etc.) have been very helpful for some pilots, who find it hard to get to sleep in strange places, and may be worth reading about or discussing with a therapist. As I have mentioned, the inability to get a good night's sleep because of too much caffeine during the trip or too much alcohol, which prevents a true restful sleep, leads to fatigue the following day. A combination of dehydration and caffeine prevents you from relaxing afterwards and makes your next trip far more fatiguing. Continuous noise is also fatiguing. The inactivity of sitting during a long, boring trip is fatiguing. Irregular hours to which the body clock is unaccustomed lead to fatigue. Going from one time zone through several other time zones, trying to get rest, and coming back also leads to fatigue. Every one of these can happen on the same trip;

some you can't control and some you can. Your hours may be difficult to change, but you certainly don't have to have those four or five cups of coffee or the "night-cap." Instead of going out with the crew before the turn-around the next day, get a good night's sleep. Don't get dehydrated, and keep in mind that your body assumes you are back home. Everyone has his own tolerances, and this is something you have to establish yourself, but you also must respect and identify those factors which lead to increased fatigue, especially those you can control.

STRESS MANAGEMENT

This is something that is poorly accepted by most people, especially flight crews. Pilots seem to feel that they are immune to the stresses of life and that they can cope with most every problem, and certainly that they should be able to single-handedly control their emotions and life's stresses. Unfortunately you are human like everybody else, and your ability to cope with these stresses will begin to show up insidiously in other problems such as poor weight control, increased blood pressure, and pulse, unexplained headaches, fatigue, inability to do your job, flunking check rides, etc. The only comment that I want to make is that despite the skepticism about counseling by psychologists and psychiatrists, you may consider talking out your problems with somebody who can be objective and trained in analyzing your real problems—which may be different than those you appear to have. This counseling is *not* disqualifying to the FAA. In fact, your inability to cope with your stresses is more of a danger to flying than seeking help from a professional who can relieve the stresses or help you to cope with them.

FIRST AID ON TRIPS

Ear Blocks

We have discussed this in Chapter 4 and I refer you to the section on hearing.

Constipation

This is almost invariably related to inactivity, dehydration and the lack of bulk in your diet. This can usually be corrected by doing the same things that we have talked about before. Maintaining a good fluid intake, eating lots of "rabbit foods" such as celery, carrots, apples, etc. In addition, you might try to establish more of a habit of following the "urge" rather than waiting until the end of the trip.

Diarrhea

This is often a result of the flu or indiscrete eating, and often there's very little you can do about it. The main thing you can do if you are caught with this in the middle of a trip is to stay away from all solid foods and stay mainly with liquids until you can return home. Trying to treat it further than that by yourself may be masking a more serious medical problem.

Rectal Itching

Sitting for long hours often creates that very uncomfortable irritation which may or may not be hemorrhoids. More than likely it is a combination of sweating, hygiene and poor-quality toilet paper in the terminals. A product called "Tucks" has been found to be very beneficial; carry it along in your flight bag. You should use these to supplement hygiene while on the trip and to even put a fresh pad right against the rectum if you are particularly uncomfortable. If the itching persists, you may have a very common "yeast" infection for which you should be seen by a doctor. In any case, persistent rectal itching is not something you should have to tolerate. It can be controlled.

Sore Legs

This almost invariably is related to inactivity and poor venous circulation. There are several tips such as pushing and then relaxing both feet against the rudder pedals, wiggling your toes frequently, and getting up and moving around. Some people have poorer circulation than others, and are therefore bothered more. Wearing good support hose (those that you buy in a drug store) also is beneficial. If you happen to notice sore leg symptoms, the chances are that they will only get worse and lead to more serious varicose veins. Don't just put up with the discomfort. Try to do something about it to correct the problem.

Colds and Flu

Obviously one shouldn't fly under these conditions, but sometimes you are caught with this in the middle of a trip. If there is any way that you can, ground yourself and dead-head back. If you can't, stay away from medications because they will only make things worse. Follow a liquid diet and pass responsibilities to your colleagues. You can't cure it, and you can't take away the symptoms without creating more symptoms, despite what the ads say.

RETIREMENT

Finally, I would like to make a few comments about retirement, whether you have to retire medically or you are forced to at age 60. This is something that very few pilots think about, especially in terms of preparation. If you are fortunate enough to maintain your health until you are age 60, what are you going to do with this good health? What happens if you have to retire because of some medical problem that is beyond your control? It is far better *now* to have an idea of what you could do, especially since you already know you are going to have to retire at age 60. I suggest you consider some sort of income producing hobby, some sort of vocation you could always fall back on and start thinking about it now. Even if you're in your 30s, if you should happen to see a course in an adult education program that interests you, go ahead and take it instead of just thinking about it. Talk with your friends about what they're doing. Those fringe benefits of retirement pay and disability pay are not going to be the answer. The philosophy, "I've paid my dues and now I can play," just doesn't work because without meaningful activity, one falls apart. Besides, some pilots find flying less than challenging as they get older. One of the things I have found in the aviation community is that once somebody is medically retired or is retired at age 60, he is somewhat a forgotten man. Remember, you will be in that situation someday, so keep in touch with the retired and find out what they are doing. I have seen too many pilots who have been grounded unexpectedly who literally waste away because they have nothing to do. They had not planned ahead and the fact that they are grounded is too much for them to cope with.

Conclusion

When anyone is confronted with an unexpected illness or unsuspected serious disease, that person will understandably use different methods of "denial" initially, such as putting off seeking help, second-guessing the diagnosis and therapy of the doctor, and looking for any way out, even to the extent of going to "quacks" for therapy. The professional pilot who has a career at stake uses this denial process even more frequently, even to the point of sacrificing his health to maintain his career as a pilot. This is understandable but unrealistic. If, in fact, you have a disorder that will keep you from flying, the sooner you find out about it, the sooner you can look for an alternative career and then more easily accept the fate of your illness. Unfortunately most professional pilots consider flying to be the *only* way to work, and they plan their professional lives accordingly. As a result, a pilot who hasn't even considered a second career cannot and often will not accept a disqualifying illness—or a mandatory age 60 retirement. Accept the fact that you have smaller chance of fulfilling your dream of being a professional pilot than anyone else—for non-pilots can return to work after a heart attack or the day after their 60th birthday. Being prepared for these odds of losing your medical certificate will make you less defensive about that unexpected disqualifying illness and allow your doctor the opportunity to help you with all your careers, *including* flying.

Nothing that I have said in this chapter has been anything new to you, but I do want you to put these matters in proper perspective. Hopefully, being a healthy, safe pilot with a current medical certificate is more important than those abuses I have described. Any one of these problems alone probably is insignificant. If you start combining them, then you are going to run into trouble. Very few pilots are grounded for reasons that were caused *solely* by events beyond their control. Documentation of your health and keeping your health is one thing, but being healthy while you are flying is yet another. In fact, you have four standards of health: The first is that state of health that *you* desire. The second is that state of health that your doctor desires. The third is that state of health that the FAA requires to certify you. The fourth is that state of health that you must have *while you are flying*. All four could be different and have different consequences on you and your career.

Appendix I
PART 67 of Federal Air Regulations

The following is a definition of the regulations that your AME and the FAA will use to pass judgment on you and your medical certificate. The actual regulations are in caps and my interpretation and explanation is in upper and lower case type.

FAR 67.13 FIRST CLASS MEDICAL CERTIFICATE
(a) TO BE ELIGIBLE FOR A FIRST CLASS MEDICAL CERTIFICATE, AN APPLICANT MUST MEET THE REQUIREMENTS OF PARAGRAPHS B THROUGH F OF THIS SECTION:
(b) EYES:
  (1) DISTANT VISUAL ACUITY OF 20/20 OR BETTER IN EACH EYE SEPARATELY WITHOUT CORRECTION: (Each eye must have perfect vision or meet the next requirement:) OR OF AT LEAST 20/100 IN EACH EYE SEPARATELY CORRECTED TO 20/20 OR BETTER WITH CORRECTIVE LENSES IN WHICH CASE THE APPLICANT MAY BE QUALIFIED ONLY ON THE CONDITION THAT HE WEARS THOSE GLASSES WHILE EXERCISING THE PRIVILEGES OF HIS AIRMAN CERTIFICATE.
  If your vision is no worse than 20/100 in either eye, then it must be corrected to perfect vision by corrective lenses—contact or frame—in order to meet this criterion. Uncorrected vision in either eye of worse than 20/100 requires further evaluation by your *eye* doctor in order to be accepted by the FAA.
  (2) NEAR VISION OF AT LEAST 20/40 IN EACH EYE EITHER WITH OR WITHOUT CORRECTION.
  This also means that if you have near vision worse than 20/40 it would be acceptable as long as it is corrected to 20/40 or better.

Pilot's Manual of Medical Certification

(3) **NORMAL COLOR VISION**

When taking the color vision test commonly used, you must not miss more than four out of the fifteen plates (or colored numbers). In other words, if you miss five or more, you do not pass. However, color vision is a very subjective sense and often a more sophisticated test, such as one using actual lights, will allow a pilot to pass the color vision test without the necessity of a waiver, even without passing the commonly used test booklet.

(4) **NORMAL FIELDS OF VISION**

You should be able to see more than that which is just straight ahead of you. Having normal fields of vision means having the ability to see a complete view, central and peripheral, with the exception of your natural blindspot in each eye. This is tested by various methods, such as watching the medical examiner's finger as he moves it from outside the field inward until it reaches your sight, or by the use of a pointer against a black screen while you are looking straight ahead, or by the use of illuminated patterns of dots flashed momentarily before you.

(5) **NO ACUTE OR CHRONIC PATHOLOGICAL CONDITION OF EITHER EYE OR ADENEXAE THAT MIGHT INTERFERE WITH PROPER FUNCTION, MIGHT PROGRESS TO THAT DEGREE OR MIGHT BE AGGRAVATED BY FLYING.**

You cannot have any ailment that would interfere with the function of your eye(s) which would limit your ability as a safe crew member. This could mean anything such as pinkeye, injury, cataracts, etc. Some of these disorders are transient and will resolve in time, others are progressive.

(6) **BIFOVEAL FIXATION AND VERGENCEPHORIA RELATIONSHIP SUFFICIENT TO PREVENT A BREAK IN FUSION UNDER CONDITIONS THAT MAY REASONABLY OCCUR IN PERFORMING AIRMAN DUTIES.**

This is a bunch of fancy words which mean simply that you need two eyes that look at the same object without seeing a double image. This usually is checked by having you look into a vision-testing instrument and tell the examiner over which line a dot falls. This then defines your ability to fuse your two eyes on one object.

(c) **EAR, NOSE, THROAT, AND EQUILIBRIUM:**

(1) ABILITY TO —

(i) HEAR THE WHISPERED VOICE AT A DISTANCE

Appendix I

OF AT LEAST 20 FEET WITH EACH EAR SEPARATELY; OR

(ii) DEMONSTRATE A HEARING ACUITY OF AT LEAST 50 PERCENT OF NORMAL IN EACH EAR THROUGHOUT THE EFFECTIVE SPEECH AND RADIO RANGE AS SHOWN BY A STANDARD AUDIOMETER.

The whispered voice has been used for years but is not an accurate test of your hearing ability. The use of an audiometer for first class physicals is expected by the FAA. In terms of numbers, if you have a hearing loss greater than 40 db for 500 and 35 db in the range of 1000, and 2000 cycles per second, (the usual voice range), you would not pass the initial examination. Keep in mind, however, that this is already quite a hearing loss. Most hearing deficiencies in the *higher* frequencies are a direct result of being exposed to noise.

(2) NO ACUTE OR CHRONIC DISEASE OF THE MIDDLE OR INTERNAL EAR
(3) NO DISEASE OF THE MASTOID
(4) NO UNHEALED (UNCLOSED) PERFORATION OF THE EARDRUM
(5) NO DISEASE OR MALFORMATION OF THE NOSE OR THROAT THAT MIGHT *INTERFERE WITH* (OR BE AGGRAVATED BY) FLYING
(6) NO DISTURBANCE IN EQUILIBRIUM

These are all self-explanatory. You should keep in mind that these all are essential senses that must be used while flying. The actual act of flying can aggravate many of these. Therefore, a minor problem with the ear at ground level would be extremely distracting at an elevated cabin altitude or during a moderate aircraft maneuver.

(d) MENTAL AND NEUROLOGIC:
(1) MENTAL
(i) NO ESTABLISHED MEDICAL HISTORY OR CLINICAL DIAGNOSIS OF ANY OF THE FOLLOWING:
(a) A PERSONALITY DISORDER THAT IS SEVERE ENOUGH TO HAVE REPEATEDLY MANIFESTED ITSELF BY OVERT ACTS.
(b) A PSYCHOSIS.
(c) ALCOHOLISM, UNLESS THERE IS ESTABLISHED CLINICAL EVIDENCE, SATISFACTORY TO THE FEDERAL AIR SURGEON, OF

RECOVERY, INCLUDING SUSTAINED TOTAL ABSTINENCE FROM ALCOHOL FOR NOT LESS THAN THE PRECEDING 2 YEARS. AS USED IN THIS SECTION, "ALCOHOLISM" MEANS A CONDITION IN WHICH A PERSON'S INTAKE OF ALCOHOL IS GREAT ENOUGH TO DAMAGE PHYSICAL HEALTH OR PERSONAL OR SOCIAL FUNCTIONING, OR WHEN ALCOHOL HAS BECOME A PREREQUISITE TO NORMAL FUNCTIONING.
  (d) DRUG DEPENDENCE.
   These all have been previously described as part of the nine mandatory disqualifications.
 (ii) NO OTHER PERSONALITY DISORDER, NEUROSIS, OR MENTAL CONDITION THAT THE FEDERAL AIR SURGEON FINDS—
  (a) MAKES THE APPLICANT UNABLE TO SAFELY PERFORM THE DUTIES OR EXERCISE THE PRIVILEGES OF THE AIRMAN CERTIFICATE THAT HE HOLDS OR FOR WHICH HE IS APPLYING; OR
  (b) MAY REASONABLY BE EXPECTED, WITHIN TWO YEARS AFTER THE FINDING, TO MAKE HIM UNABLE TO PERFORM THOSE DUTIES OR EXERCISE THOSE PRIVILEGES; AND THE FINDINGS ARE BASED ON THE CASE HISTORY AND APPROPRIATE, QUALIFIED, MEDICAL JUDGEMENT RELATING TO THE CONDITION INVOLVED.
   This is a very subjective regulation, difficult to clearly define, diagnose, and document. This could be categorized as a "catch all" for *any* psychological problem that would interfere with safe flying.

(2) NEUROLOGIC
  (i) NO ESTABLISHED MEDICAL HISTORY OR CLINICAL DIAGNOSIS OF EITHER OF THE FOLLOWING:
   (a) EPILEPSY
   (b) A DISTURBANCE OF CONSCIOUSNESS WITHOUT SATISFACTORY MEDICAL EXPLANATION OF THE CAUSE.
  (ii) NO OTHER CONVULSIVE DISORDER, DISTURBANCE OF CONSCIOUSNESS, OR NEUROLOGIC

Appendix I

CONDITION THAT THE FEDERAL AIR SURGEON FINDS—
- (a) MAKES THE APPLICANT UNABLE TO SAFELY PERFORM THE DUTIES OR EXERCISE THE PRIVILEGES OF THE AIRMAN CERTIFICATE THAT HE HOLDS OR FOR WHICH HE IS APPLYING; OR
- (b) MAY REASONABLY BE EXPECTED, WITHIN TWO YEARS AFTER THE FINDING, TO MAKE HIM UNABLE TO PERFORM THOSE DUTIES OR EXERCISE THOSE PRIVILEGES; AND THE FINDINGS ARE BASED ON THE CASE HISTORY AND APPROPRIATE, QUALIFIED, MEDICAL JUDGEMENT RELATING TO THE CONDITION INVOLVED.

This is basically the same as described earlier in the mandatory denials. Keep in mind that this allows the Federal Air Surgeon to pass judgment, based on the information provided him, as to whether your abnormal neurological condition would interfere with the safety of flying. We discuss elsewhere in the book how the medical profession interprets and judges medical data to determine whether or not a pilot is safe to fly.

(e) CARDIOVASCULAR:
  (1) NO ESTABLISHED MEDICAL HISTORY OR CLINICAL DIAGNOSIS OF—
     (i) MYOCARDIAL INFARCTION;
     (ii) ANGINA PECTORIS; OR
     (iii) CORONARY HEART DISEASE THAT HAS REQUIRED TREATMENT OR, IF UNTREATED, THAT HAS BEEN SYMPTOMATIC OR CLINICALLY SIGNIFICANT.
  (2) IF THE APPLICANT HAS PASSED HIS THIRTY-FIFTH BIRTHDAY BUT NOT HIS FORTIETH, HE MUST, ON THE FIRST EXAMINATION AFTER HIS THIRTY-FIFTH BIRTHDAY, SHOW AN ABSENCE OF MYOCARDIAL INFARCTION ON ELECTROCARDIOGRAPHIC EXAMINATION.

  Note that the purpose of the EKG is to prove the *absence of an MI*, not to prove that you have a healthy heart.

  (3) IF THE APPLICANT HAS PASSED HIS FORIETH BIRTHDAY, HE MUST ANNUALLY SHOW AN ABSENCE OF MYOCARDIAL INFARCTION ON ELECTROCARDIOGRAPHIC EXAMINATION.

(4) UNLESS THE ADJUSTED MAXIMUM READINGS APPLY, THE APPLICANT'S RECLINING BLOOD PRESSURE MAY NOT BE MORE THAN THE MAXIMUM READING FOR HIS AGE GROUP IN THE FOLLOWING TABLE:

Age Group	Maximum readings (reclining blood pressure in mm) Systolic	Diastolic	Adjusted maximum Readings (reclining blood pressure in mm)[1] Systolic	Diastolic
20-29	140	88	—	—
30-39	145	92	155	98
40-49	155	96	165	100
50 and over	160	98	170	100

[1]For an applicant at least 30 years of age whose reclining blood pressure is more than the maximum reading of his age group and whose cardiac and kidney conditions, after complete cardiovascular examination, are found to be normal.

Note that there are two key words here. One is the *"adjusted"* maximum reading, which applies if you have had a complete cardiovascular evaluation and everything has been found to be within acceptable limits, except, of course, your blood pressure readings. In this case, the acceptable limits of your blood pressure are higher and thus accepted by the FAA. The other key word is *reclining*. The regulation refers to your reclining blood pressure, not sitting.

(5) IF THE APPLICANT IS AT LEAST 40 YEARS OF AGE, HE MUST SHOW A DEGREE OF CIRCULATORY EFFICIENCY THAT IS COMPATIBLE WITH THE SAFE OPERATION OF AIRCRAFT AT HIGH ALTITUDES.

This is another one of those catch-all categories which include many diseases and medical abnormalities dealing with your general circulation, especially your heart. The key here is that, again, a medical problem *you* feel is not significant or symptomatic while on ground may become a very risky problem at higher altitudes with less oxygen, humidity, etc.

Appendix I

(f) GENERAL MEDICAL CONDITION:
  (1) NO ESTABLISHED MEDICAL HISTORY OR CLINICAL DIAGNOSIS OF DIABETES MELLITUS THAT REQUIRES INSULIN OR ANY OTHER HYPOGLYCEMIC DRUG FOR CONTROL.

  This was described earlier under one of the mandatory denials.

  (2) NO OTHER ORGANIC, FUNCTIONAL, OR STRUCTURAL DISEASE, DEFECT, OR LIMITATION THAT THE FEDERAL AIR SURGEON FINDS—
    (i) MAKES THE APPLICANT UNABLE TO SAFELY PERFORM THE DUTIES OR EXERCISE THE PRIVILEGES OF THE AIRMAN CERTIFICATE THAT HE HOLDS OR FOR WHICH HE IS APPLYING; OR
    (ii) MAY REASONABLY BE EXPECTED, WITHIN TWO YEARS AFTER THE FINDING, TO MAKE HIM UNABLE TO PERFORM THOSE DUTIES OR EXERCISE THOSE PRIVILEGES; AND THE FINDINGS ARE BASED ON THE CASE HISTORY AND APPROPRIATE, QUALIFIED, MEDICAL JUDGMENT RELATING TO THE CONDITION INVOLVED.

    This is the "catch-all" of them all and includes *any* medical problem considered detrimental to safe flying. You can look at it in two ways: either that it allows the FAA to ground you for the slightest problem or that it, by the same token, allows the Federal Air Surgeon to be flexible in his judgement for a *real* medical problem and allow you to *continue* flying if he feels that it would not interfere with your responsibilities as an aircrew member.

(g) AN APPLICANT WHO DOES NOT MEET THE PROVISIONS OF PARAGRAPHS (B) THROUGH (F) OF THIS SECTION MAY APPLY FOR THE DISCRETIONARY ISSUANCE OF A CERTIFICATE UNDER § 67.19.

  This regulation means that practically all disorders are potentially certifiable if the condition does not compromise safe flying.

§ 67.19 SPECIAL ISSUE OF MEDICAL CERTIFICATES.
(a) AT THE DISCRETION OF THE FEDERAL AIR SURGEON, A MEDICAL CERTIFICATE MAY BE ISSUED TO AN APPLICANT WHO DOES NOT MEET THE APPLICABLE PROVISIONS OF §§ 67.13, 67.15, or § 67.17 IF THE APPLICANT SHOWS TO THE SATISFACTION OF THE FEDERAL AIR

SURGEON THAT THE DUTIES AUTHORIZED BY THE CLASS OF MEDICAL CERTIFICATE APPLIED FOR CAN BE PERFORMED WITHOUT ENDANGERING AIR COMMERCE DURING THE PERIOD IN WHICH THE CERTIFICATE WOULD BE IN FORCE. THE FEDERAL AIR SURGEON MAY AUTHORIZE A SPECIAL MEDICAL FLIGHT TEST, PRACTICAL TEST, OR MEDICAL EVALUATION FOR THIS PURPOSE.

(b) THE FEDERAL AIR SURGEON MAY CONSIDER THE APPLICANT'S OPERATIONAL EXPERIENCE AND ANY MEDICAL FACTS THAT MAY AFFECT THE ABILITY OF THE APPLICANT TO PERFORM AIRMAN DUTIES INCLUDING:

(1) THE COMBINED EFFECT ON THE APPLICANT OF FAILURE TO MEET MORE THAN ONE REQUIREMENT OF THIS PART; AND

(2) THE PROGNOSIS DERIVED FROM PROFESSIONAL CONSIDERATION OF ALL AVAILABLE INFORMATION REGARDING THE AIRMAN.

(c) IN DETERMINING WHETHER THE SPECIAL ISSUANCE OF A THIRD-CLASS MEDICAL CERTIFICATE SHOULD BE MADE TO AN APPLICANT, THE FEDERAL AIR SURGEON CONSIDERS THE FREEDOM OF AN AIRMAN, EXERCISING THE PRIVILEGES OF A PRIVATE PILOT CERTIFICATE, TO ACCEPT REASONABLE RISKS TO HIS OR HER PERSON AND PROPERTY THAT ARE NOT ACCEPTABLE IN THE EXERCISE OF COMMERCIAL OR AIRLINE TRANSPORT PRIVILEGES, AND, AT THE SAME TIME, CONSIDERS THE NEED TO PROTECT THE PUBLIC SAFETY OF PERSONS AND PROPERTY IN OTHER AIRCRAFT AND ON THE GROUND.

(d) IN ISSUING A MEDICAL CERTIFICATE UNDER THIS SECTION, THE FEDERAL AIR SURGEON MAY DO ANY OR ALL OF THE FOLLOWING:

(1) LIMIT THE DURATION OF THE CERTIFICATE.

(2) CONDITION THE CONTINUED EFFECT OF THE CERTIFICATE ON THE RESULTS OF SUBSEQUENT MEDICAL TESTS, EXAMINATIONS, OR EVALUATIONS.

(3) IMPOSE ANY OPERATIONAL LIMITATION ON THE CERTIFICATE NEEDED FOR SAFETY.

(4) CONDITION THE CONTINUED EFFECT OF A SECOND- OR THIRD-CLASS MEDICAL CERTIFICATE ON COMPLIANCE WITH A STATEMENT OF FUNC-

Appendix I

TIONAL LIMITATIONS ISSUED TO THE APPLICANT IN COORDINATION WITH THE DIRECTOR OF FLIGHT OPERATIONS OR THE DIRECTOR'S DESIGNEE.

(e) AN APPLICANT WHO HAS BEEN ISSUED A MEDICAL CERTIFICATE UNDER THIS SECTION BASED ON A SPECIAL MEDICAL FLIGHT OR PRACTICAL TEST NEED NOT TAKE THE TEST AGAIN DURING LATER PHYSICAL EXAMINATIONS UNLESS THE FEDERAL AIR SURGEON DETERMINES THAT THE PHYSICAL DEFICIENCY HAS BECOME ENOUGH MORE PRONOUNCED TO REQUIRE ANOTHER SPECIAL MEDICAL FLIGHT OR PRACTICAL TEST.

(f) THE AUTHORITY OF THE FEDERAL AIR SURGEON UNDER THIS SECTION IS ALSO EXERCISED BY THE CHIEF, AEROMEDICAL CERTIFICATION BRANCH, CIVIL AEROMEDICAL INSTITUTE, AND EACH REGIONAL FLIGHT SURGEON.

(This regulation is self explanatory, but comments are made in chapter three).

Appendix II
Conditions for which the Medical Certificate Will Be Denied or Deferred

A listing of the conditions as found in the *Guide for Aviation Medical Examiners.*

The conditions for which a certificate will be denied or deferred are categorized by the different body functions, starting with the head and working down. In addition, they follow the pattern set forth on the back of form 8500-8. One point to remember is that many of these problems are of the transient nature, such as an infection, and with appropriate therapy will go away. While you have the infection you should not be flying and you would be temporarily "disqualified" if you were to take your examination while you had the infection. However, as soon as the infection is gone, that is, there is an *absence* of the infection, you would be legal to fly and would be able to pass your physical if you took it at that time. In the following cases, we are *not* talking about a *history* of a specific medical problem (as defined in the nine mandatory denials), but rather whether or not you *presently* have a problem. For example: On Monday, you take your FAA physical and pass it. On Tuesday, you develop a middle ear infection. On this same Tuesday you would not be qualified to fly per FAR 61.53 and 67.13(c)(2). *If* you had taken your FAA exam on that Tuesday instead of Monday, you wouldn't have passed but would have been "grounded." If you waited until the *following* Monday to take your FAA exam and the ear infection was gone, you would then pass your physical.

The "Guide" in use until recently was dated 1970. A new guide, which *medically* is basically the same, has been published by the FAA and should be in the hands of most AMEs by March 1982. The improvement in the current guide is a more clearly defined protocol for the AME to follow—i.e. a better "guide" for your AME to help you if you have a problem. In other words, your AME now has the *tools* to

Appendix II

assist you, yet he may still elect to "pass the buck" to the FAA as described in the book. It remains, therefore, important for you to be familiar with this "Guide" plus the material in the book so that you can advise your AME as to what you expect from him.

Now let's consider the pertinent medical items that could create problems in your medical certification. You then will understand why you shouldn't fly with any of these problems. The items in capital letters are taken directly out of the AME's guide. (Although some of the wordage is from the older 1970 Guide, the intent is the same.) The sentences in upper and lower case letters are my explanations. Any specific problems you may have should be discussed with a flight surgeon for adequate explanation.

ITEM 25 — HEAD, FACE, NECK, AND SCALP

(a) FISTULA OF NECK, EITHER CONGENITAL OR ACQUIRED, TO INCLUDE TRACHEOTOMY.

This means that you cannot have a hole (fistula) in the neck which could interfere with normal function. A tracheotomy, obviously, is not compatible with flying as an aircrew member, but even more important is that the *reason* itself for the tracheotomy probably is more hazardous.

(b) LOSS OF BONY SUBSTANCE INVOLVING THE TWO TABLES OF THE CRANIAL VAULT.

Missing any part of the skull is not for pilots!

(c) CLASSES I AND II ONLY: DEFORMITIES OF FACE OR HEAD WHICH WOULD INTERFERE WITH WEARING AND PROPER FITTING OF ANY OXYGEN MASK.

ITEM 26 — NOSE

(a) EVIDENCE OF ALLERGIC RHINITIS.

Allergic rhinitis is hayfever. This mainly deals with the nose being so congested from the hayfever that you cannot breathe properly, which can create problems at usual cabin altitudes and during descents. Hayfever also can lead to additional breathing disorders.

(b) MALFORMATION WHICH WOULD PREVENT NASAL RESPIRATION.

A pilot should be able to breathe *through* the nose (not solely through the mouth). A malformation could interfere with this normal breathing. This malformation also means the potential inability to "clear your ears" (valsalva).

(c) OBSTRUCTION OF SINUS OSTIA, INCLUDING POLYPS, WHICH WOULD BE LIKELY TO RESULT IN COMPLETE CLOSURE UNDER CONDITIONS TO WHICH AIRMEN ARE EXPOSED.

"Sinus Ostia" are the openings from inside your nose to your sinuses in your head. Obviously, if they are obstructed you may develop a sinus block, especially during a descent. The resulting pain is more than just distracting to a pilot. Ask someone who has had one!

ITEM 27—SINUSES
(a) SINUSITIS:
  (1) ACUTE
      This Sinusitis is a transient sinus infection, as experienced during a "cold." Again, the inability to equalize the pressure in your ears and sinuses (valsalva) is the reason you should *not* fly with a cold or acute sinusitis.
  (2) CHRONIC, PURULENT—CONFIRMED BY X-RAY
      Some people have a chronic (ongoing) sinus infection that does not respond to usual therapy. In addition to being a risk in flying, these people just don't feel good anyway and usually are under the care of a doctor.
(b) TUMOR

The presence of any tumor anywhere in the body is subject to suspicion until proven that it does not interfere with flying.

An explanation of tumors in general may be appropriate at this time. A "tumor" is any lump of tissue in the body that is not supposed to be there. If it becomes infected, like a boil, it becomes uncomfortable or painful. If it interferes with the normal function of your body, then the tumor is not compatible with flying until it is removed. A tumor that continues to grow or to spread, like a malignant tumor, obviously is not compatible with flying. The problem with a malignant tumor is not that it is malignant (which means it spreads), but that it is spreading to other parts of the body and thereby interfering with or stopping the function of various vital organs. In other words, a tumor like a common lipoma (a fatty growth which is benign and usually found in the skin) is of no *medical* consequence unless, for instance, it is at the belt line and continues to become aggravated by your belt or by the seat belt. These often do become inflamed or infected and then become quite painful and distracting. A malignant tumor, on the other hand, such as cancer of the bowel, in addition to interfering with normal bowel function, begins to invade other functions of the body and can create a general debilitation and weakness so that the pilot is just too sick to fly. Although the pilot with these "tumors" may feel all right, the issue is how these "tumors" affect him *while he is flying*. Experience has shown that those tumors not compatible with flying are, in fact, dangerous to that pilot even though he may not be personally aware of any symptoms or potential danger.

Appendix II

ITEM 28 — MOUTH AND THROAT
(a) PALATE: EXTENSIVE ADHESION OF THE SOFT PALATE TO THE PHARYNX.

An "adhesion" is a fibrous attachment of the soft palate to your breathing passages which prevents normal breathing patterns. At altitude, wearing a mask, or under stressful situations, this is a potentially dangerous disorder.

(b) ANY MALFORMATION OR CONDITION, INCLUDING STUTTERING, WHICH WOULD IMPAIR VOICE COMMUNICATION.

ITEM 29 — EARS, GENERAL
(a) INNER EAR: ACUTE OR CHRONIC DISEASE WHICH MAY DISTURB EQUILIBRIUM.

A disturbance in equilibrium is, in this case, the same as the vertigo or dizziness one would experience in moving the head up, down, or sideways during a steep turn. Even under normal circumstances this is very disabling. Any further disease of the "balance-maintaining mechanism" adds to this already disabling condition. A viral labyrinthitis, which many of us have experienced at one time or another, is the more common entity in this category and can lead to extreme vertigo.

(b) MASTOIDS:
   (1) MASTOIDITIS, ACUTE OR CHRONIC.
   (2) MASTOID FISTULA.

The mastoid is a form of sinus located in the bony protrusion just behind the external ear and once was a common location for infection. Anyone with a mastoid infection was quite ill and would not feel like driving a car, much less flying a plane. With the advent of antibiotics, however, mastoid infections are uncommon.

(c) MIDDLE EAR:
   (1) OTITIS MEDIA, SEROUS OR SUPPURATIVE, ACUTE OR CHRONIC.

Otitis media is a middle ear infection inside the eardrum which most of us have experienced at one time or another. This was more common when you were a child, but as a pilot or as a scuba diver, the infection can lead to a severe ear block.

   (2) IMPAIRED AERATION

Congestion can easily block the eustachian tube and prevent you from doing a "valsalva" maneuver, that is equalizing your middle ear air pressure by holding your nose and blowing against it. This painful block is often experienced on descents when you have a cold. A doctor can see the movement of your ear drum when you do a valsalva maneuver and it is through this technique that he determines if you are able to clear your ears. Aeration means the ability of the eustachian tube to maintain equal air pressure on both sides of the ear drum.

(d) OUTER EAR:
  (1) OTITIS EXTERNA WHICH MAY PROGRESS TO IMPAIR HEARING OR BECOME INCAPACITATING

  Otitis externa is an infection of the outer ear *canal*. Those who have experienced this know that it is very painful. Because of the swelling, it decreases your hearing.

  (2) IMPACTED CERUMEN UNTIL REMOVED.

  This implies that the packed-in ear wax prevents you from hearing well until it is removed, as though you were wearing an ear plug.

ITEM 30 — EAR DRUMS

(a) ANY PERFORATION ASSOCIATED WITH ACTIVE INFECTION

The key in this disorder is whether there is an *active infection* in progress. A perforation after an infection has cleared is acceptable as long as it doesn't interfere with hearing. However any perforation increases your risk of infection.

(b) SEVERE RETRACTION.

Severe retraction (a deformed eardrum) results when there has been sufficient damage done by an old infection or other disease in inhibit free movement of the eardrum. This would show up mainly in your inability to pass an audiogram or hearing test.

ITEM 31 — EYES, GENERAL

(a) ACUTE OR CHRONIC PATHOLOGICAL CONDITION OF EITHER EYE OR ADNEXA WHICH MAY INTERFERE WITH ITS PROPER FUNCTION, MAY PROGRESS TO THAT DEGREE, OR MAY BE AGGRAVATED BY FLYING.

This is self explanatory. It means that any condition that would interfere with the use of your eyes and their adjacent parts, especially while flying, is not compatible with safety.

(b) NYSTAGMUS WITH BOTH EYES FIXING.

"Nystagmus" is an involuntary movement of the eyes, very uncommon, and usually associated with *other* disease processes. It is the other disease processes that usually are disqualifying, although the "nystagmus" is what the doctor will note first on his exam.

(c) STRABISMUS.

Strabismus (cross-eyes) prevents a pilot from seeing an object

Appendix II

as a single image and the pilot usually perceives this as double vision, especially when tired, fatigued, or at altitude.

(d) PTOSIS WHICH INTERFERES WITH VISION.

Ptosis means lowering or drooping of the eyelid and obviously if it interferes with your vision, it is not a safe way to fly.

(e) EXOPHTHALMOS: UNILATERAL OR BILATERAL.

This is an abnormal protrusion of the eyeball. It can be either one eye or both and is usually associated with other disease processes such as thyroid disorders. Again, as long as the vision is all right, the presence of the exophthalmos *by itself* doesn't create a problem, but is an indication of another disease going on.

(f) GLAUCOMA

The presence of glaucoma means that destruction of the retina is taking place, which also means that the vision is deteriorating. Glaucoma which is controlled and is not affecting vision is certifiable.

(g) APHAKIA: UNILATERAL OR BILATERAL

This is the lack of a lens within the eyeball for any reason. You can't focus without a lens.

ITEM 32 – OPTHALMOSCOPIC

In an opthalmoscopic examination, the doc looks into your eye with a special flashlight and will often "dial" in different lenses while he is looking. He uses a small hand-held instrument which is not the same as that used by a doctor checking your vision for glasses. Instead, the doctor actually looks *inside* the eyeball so that he can see the blood vessels, nerves, and the retina. It is the only place on the body that a doctor can see these blood vessels and nerves not covered by skin.

(a) CHORIORETINITIS IF ACTIVE OR LIKELY TO RECUR.

An inflammation (redness or irritation) of the inside of the eyeball, including the retina, which results in blurred vision even with glasses.

(b) CATARACT.

A "clouding over" of the lens within the eyeball which prevents passage of light.

(c) RETINAL EXUDATE, HEMORRHAGE, OR EDEMA.
(d) DETACHMENT OF RETINA OR EVIDENCE OF SURGERY FOR CORRECTION OF DETACHMENT.
(e) INFLAMMATORY DISEASE OF THE RETINA, UVEA OR OTHER STRUCTURES WITHIN THE GLOBE; IF ACTIVE, IF IN A STATE LIKELY TO RECUR, OR IF LIKELY TO PRODUCE SIGNIFICANT INTERFERENCE WITH VISUAL FUNCTION.
(f) RETINITIS PIGMENTOSA

These are all diseases of the retina, the picture-taking mechanism of the eye, all of which lead to inadequate, blurred, or disruptive vision, none of which is compatible with safe flying.

(g) PAPILLEDEMA

This is a swelling of the optic nerve *inside* the eye. It is found only by the opthalmoscope and is usually suggestive of some *other* medical problem such as head trauma and diseases of the brain. It is not the papilledema itself that is the critical factor but that it represents something much more serious.

(h) TUMOR

As noted before, any tumor that causes any problems or interferes with proper function of the body is not compatible with safe flying.

(i) ABSENCE OF ONE OR BOTH NATURAL LENSES, REGARDLESS OF CORRECTION.

The eye is like a camera. Without a lens, you do not get a picture. The FAA will consider a waiver if the airman is able to function with one eye. This is only after additional tests and a demonstration of flying ability.

ITEM 33 — PUPILS

(a) SYNECHIAE, ANTERIOR OR POSTERIOR

The pupil controls the amount of light entering the eye, similar to the aperture in a camera. It will allow lesser or greater amounts of light depending on the intensity. Synechiae are scar tissues or adhesions of parts of the eye preventing the pupil from reacting normally.

(b) NONREACTIVE, UNTIL CAUSE DETERMINED.

If the pupil does not respond to light by contracting when a flashlight is shined into the eye, there is some other medical problem going on — usually neurological. Until the cause is found, one must assume that there is a severe medical problem.

(c) INEQUALITY, UNTIL CAUSE DETERMINED OR SATISFACTORILY EXPLAINED.

This is the same as with (b) above. If the pupils are not equal in size, it is usually secondary to some medical problem that could be serious. Until those suspicious medical problems have been ruled out, we must assume that this condition is not compatible with flying.

ITEM 34 — OCULAR MOTILITY

(a) PARALYSIS OF OCULAR MOTION IN ANY DIRECTION.
(b) ABSENCE OF CONJUGATE ALIGNMENT IN ANY QUADRANT.

Both of these conditions prevent the eyes from functioning as a team. Both eyes should be able to move in all directions and to

Appendix II

function *together* so that there are not in effect two "cameras" taking pictures of the same object and giving you a double image.
(c) INABILITY TO CONVERGE ON NEAR OBJECT

If your eyes are not able to converge on an object that is near to you, such as a book you are reading, one eye will "break away" and you will be left with vision out of only one eye. The ability of the eyes to converge decreases with age. Failure to converge at a reasonable distance, for instance one foot from the eyes, is not compatible with flying safely and reading charts and instruments unless there is no double vision.

ITEM 35 — LUNGS AND CHEST
(a) BRONCHIECTASIS, IF MORE THAN MILD.

This is only determined by a chest x-ray but sometimes it can be detected with a stethoscope. Bronchiectases is a localized area within the lung that does not expand with inspiration of air. It may be fibrous in nature, and therefore does not function as lung tissue should.

(b) EMPHYSEMA, IF OF SUFFICIENT DEGREE TO BE SYMPTOMATIC.

Emphysema is a chronic overexpansion of the lung. Emphysema at ground level may not be noticeable but could be quite severe at usual cabin altitudes.

(c) FIBROSIS, IF OF SUFFICIENT DEGREE TO INTERFERE WITH PULMONARY FUNCTION.

This is any part of the lung which has been *replaced* with fibrous tissue from any cause and therefore does not allow the lung to function properly. If it is severe enough to prevent normal pulmonary function, then it is not compatible with flying at altitude.

(d) FISTULA, BRONCHOPLEURAL, TO INCLUDE THORACOTOMY.

This is an opening between your breathing tubes and the lining of the lung — much like a bypass — which obviously would interfere with your breathing. This is virtually unheard-of in any active pilot since the cause of the fistula creates additional difficulties that preclude flying anyway.

(e) LOBECTOMY, UNTIL 6 MONTHS AFTER SURGERY AT WHICH TIME THE RESULTS OF PULMONARY FUNCTION TESTS WILL BE OBTAINED AND FORWARDED.

Our lungs are divided into several lobes or sections. If one of these lobes is removed, we normally still have enough reserve within our lungs to provide adequate pulmonary function. In other words, we normally only use a portion of our lungs when we breathe. By utilizing our reserves, we can afford to lose a lobe of

Pilot's Manual of Medical Certification

the lung without interfering with normal function. Therefore, the six-month delay is to insure healing and a return to normal pulmonary function after the removal of a lobe.

(f) PLEURA AND PLEURAL CAVITY:
   (1) ACUTE FIBRINOUS PLEURISY.
   (2) PLEURISY WITH EFFUSION.
   (3) EMPYEMA.

   All of these are diseases of the lining or covering of the lung and they prevent normal expansion of the lung and breathing. Once again, this may not be apparent at ground level, but could become quite severe at altitude. Like so many other processes, these conditions make a pilot so ill he wouldn't want to fly anyway.

(g) PNEUMOTHORAX

   This is a condition of the lung in which part of it has collapsed (air gets between the lung and chest wall) and it cannot function properly.
   (1) ARTIFICIAL, UNTIL 6 MONTHS AFTER CESSATION OR THERAPY
   (2) SPONTANEOUS, UNTIL RESOLVED AS DEMONSTRATED BY X-RAY, AND UNTIL IT IS DETERMINED THAT NO CONDITION IS PRESENT WHICH WOULD BE LIKELY TO CAUSE RECURRENCE.

   Artificial usually refers to a pneumothorax caused by trauma to the chest, such as a stabbing, gunshot, or auto accident. Spontaneous pneumothorax happens unexpectedly and without warning and it occurs without any specific external cause. It may be prompted by an existing disease, such as emphysema or tumor, or it may just happen in a seemingly healthy person.

(h) TUBERCULOSIS IN ACTIVE FORM AND UNTIL CONSIDERED ARRESTED.

   In addition to this statement, the FAA states that certain conditions must be met before recertification. Since TB is such an uncommon disease in a healthy pilot population, this will not be discussed other than to say that the FAA will recertify once the TB has been arrested. In addition, the *Guide* says "for *history* of pulmonary tuberculosis, the report will indicate the date on which the disease was considered arrested."

(i) TUMORS:
   (1) ABSCESSES, CYSTS, OR TUMORS OF LUNG, PLEURA, MEDIASTINUM, AND TUMORS OF THE BREAST.
   (2) SARCOID, IF MORE THAN MINIMAL INVOLVEMENT OR IF SYMPTOMATIC.

Appendix II

As described previously, any tumor that interferes with the function of a vital organ such as the lung is disqualifying, since the pilot will not be able to function at altitude or under stress. Sarcoid is a form of tumor in the lung and is usually discovered incidentally by an x-ray. Most cases of sarcoid resolve themselves after a period of several months and cause no residual disease or problem.

(j) MYCOTIC DISEASE WITH OR WITHOUT CAVITATION.

Mycotic disease is an airborne fungus which causes an infection in the lung. These are not usually found unless a routine chest x-ray is taken or the pilot is severely ill. Many mycotic problems do respond to therapy and time with minimal residual problems. "Cavitation" is a more serious form of the infection.

(k) OTHER DISEASES OR DEFECTS OF THE LUNGS OR CHEST WALL WHICH COULD ADVERSELY AFFECT FLYING OR ENDANGER THE INDIVIDUAL'S WELL-BEING IF PERMITTED TO FLY.

This is self-explanatory and is another "catch-all" category to include those uncommon entities which, as is stated, would affect the pilot's flying ability.

(l) ASTHMA

This is a disease whose symptoms and seriousness are subject to interpretation by the treating physician and also by the FAA physician. The FAA physician is responsible to judge whether the degree of asthma will interfere with adequate pulmonary function. A history of childhood asthma is not included in this statement, since it is well known that childhood asthma often will totally resolve itself. Since asthma is related to allergies, it can often be treated simply by avoiding the area of the country where the affected person suffers from allergies the most. If there is no asthma present, and there is no "dormant" asthma which would flare up under known circumstances, there should be no problem. However, a tendency toward asthmatic attacks, especially under known aggravating conditions or environments, is not compatible with safe flying since the asthmatic can barely breathe under those circumstances. If you take even a mild asthmatic to altitude, say six or seven thousand feet, and subject him to the stresses of flying, it could very easily precipitate an asthmatic attack which would not be symptomatic under nonflying conditions.

(m) PNEUMONECTOMY.

This is the removal of one whole lung, which would greatly compromise the pulmonary function of an airman. However, let me remind you once again that all of these conditions are subject

Pilot's Manual of Medical Certification

to review and interpretation. If the breathing function of the airman is not compromised, even at altitude, the FAA could certify him.

ITEM 36—HEART

(a) ANGINA PECTORIS OR OTHER EVIDENCE OF CORONARY HEART DISEASE.

Any evidence of coronary artery disease—angia pectoris being one form of evidence—is not compatible with safe flying. It is disqualifying until is proven there is no interference with adequate function of the heart or compromise to safe flying. If you feel this is a case of being "guilty until proven innocent," you are right. But that is exactly how all medicine is practiced.

(b) HYPERTROPHY OR DILATION OF THE HEART AS EVIDENCED BY CLINICAL EXAMINATION AND SUPPORTED BY ELCTROCARDIOGRAPHIC AND X-RAY EXAMINATION.

Hypertrophy means enlargement of the heart, and when this is seen on x-ray or on examination it usually implies some cardiac illness. This does not include, in contrast, the pilot who is a long-distance runner or someone who has developed a large heart muscle mass as a result of other exercise. Until proven otherwise, a heart that is larger than normal will be considered an indication of a more-severe problem and will be disqualifying.

(c) CONGENITAL HEART DISEASE ACCOMPANIED BY CARDIAC ENLARGEMENT, ECG ABNORMALITY, OR EVIDENCE OF INADEQUATE OXYGENATION.

By itself, congenital heart disease that is asymptomatic and creates no problems at altitude is of no concern. However, if in association with this there is an enlarged heart or any other disorder which indicates that the heart cannot work normally, then congenital heart disease becomes incompatible with safe flying. The heart could fail.

(d) PERICARDITIS, ENDOCARDITIS, OR MYOCARDITIS.

These are all infections or inflammations of parts of the heart and therefore preclude its normal function. Once again, people who have these problems probably are too ill to fly anyway.

(e) VALVULAR DISEASE OF HEART WILL BE EVALUATED IN ACCORDANCE WITH THE PROCEDURES OUTLINED IN PARAGRAPH i BELOW. CERTIFICATE WILL BE DENIED WHEN ANY OF THE FOLLOWING DIAGNOSES HAS BEEN ESTABLISHED:

1. AORTIC STENOSIS AND/OR AORTIC REGURGITATION.
2. MITRAL STENOSIS.
3. MITRAL INSUFFICIENCY.

Appendix II

These all are diseases of the valves in the heart and greatly compromise the function of the "hydraulic mechanism" of the heart. Just as you would not want to fly an aircraft that has a poorly functioning hydraulic system, you would not want to fly with a pilot who has a poorly functioning heart. Further evaluation is absolutely mandatory because there are varying degrees of severity. For example, mitral stenosis means that the mitral valve is narrow but the degree of narrowing will determine whether or not the heart is functioning adequately. Simply having a diagnosis of mitral stenosis, therefore, does not mean that you cannot fly. But if it is severe enough to interfere with flying, I don't think you or anybody else would want to fly.

(f) EVIDENCE OF CARDIAC DECOMPENSATION.

This is the same as failure of the heart and is self-explanatory. A heart that fails is not compatible with any responsible job requiring a properly functioning heart.

(g) MURMUR

A murmur is a sound that can be heard with a stethoscope and is a result of some degree of turbulence of the blood as it flows through the body's hydraulic system. Murmur is not a diagnosis of a disease but is simply a symptom of something that could be wrong. A murmur may be functional, that is, of no medical consequence, or it could represent a more serious disorder usually associated with a heart valve. A murmur is evaluated to determine its *cause*. If the cause has been determined to be inconsequential and not to interfere with normal function, then a pilot with a murmur can fly. A murmur is one of the more common causes for concern since it does require further elaboration, evaluation, and subsequent interpretation by the FAA.

(h) ARRHYTHMIA

Arrhythmia is a short way to say that the heart is not beating in a regular pattern or rhythm. An occasional skipped or extra beat, if known to be benign, is of no consequence. However, most arrhythmias that are not explained are of medical significance. They can lead to a far more serious rhythm problem that severely compromises the ability of the heart to function properly or they can lead to complete failure of the heart. Relate this to a hydraulic system: If the pump isn't working properly, nothing else will work.

ITEM 37 — VASCULAR SYSTEM

(a) BLOOD AND BLOOD-FORMING TISSUE DISEASE:
   (1) ANEMIA WHEN THE HEMOGLOBIN IS LOWER THAN 12 g./100 cc. BLOOD

Keep in mind that while you may be able to function quite adequately at sea level, at altitude the problem will be compounded because the oxygen to be carried is more sparse than at sea level. Without enough blood or hemoglobin to carry this shortened supply of oxygen, you'll be in trouble. In other words, the efficiency of the "fuel supply" system is greatly compromised.

(2) POLYCYTHEMIA

This is an abnormality of the blood in which there is too much hemoglobin, too many red blood cells. It is a common finding in people who live at high altitudes, as it is the body's way of compensating for the smaller amount of oxygen available to breathe. At sea level, however, these people have problems because their blood becomes very sluggish and inefficient.

(3) LEUKEMIA AND OTHER PROGRESSIVE DISEASES OF THE RETICULOENDOTHELIAL SYSTEM.

Leukemia is like cancer of the blood cells and is the same as any other cancer. It's a bad disease.

(4) HEMOPHILIA

This is the inability of your blood clotting system to function. With hemophilia, a simple bump or scratch could become a major medical problem. If you were to bump your shin bone as you get into your seat, you could become a medical emergency in a matter of minutes because of the hemorrhaging inside your leg.

(5) OTHER DISEASE OF THE BLOOD OR BLOODFORMING TISSUES WHICH COULD ADVERSELY AFFECT PERFORMANCE OF AIRMAN DUTIES.

Once again, the key part of this phrase is "any medical problem that could adversely affect the performance of airman duties." This is a matter of common sense, but not one for the crewmember to judge unless he is well versed and trained in the risk factors for specific medical problems.

(b) PERIPHERAL VASCULAR DISEASE

This refers to diseases of the arteries and veins in the arms and legs which interfere with proper function. This not only is dangerous, particularly with changes in temperature and altitude, but is extremely painful.

(1) INTERMITTENT CLAUDICATION.
(2) BUERGER'S DISEASE.
(3) RAYNAUD'S DISEASE, OR PHENOMENON.

These are all diseases which involve the arteries and the veins and severly inhibit adequate blood flow. The analogy

Appendix II

here would be a narrowing in part of your airplane's hydraulic system somewhere down the line.

(4) THROMBOPHLEBITIS, OR PHLEBOTHROMBOSIS.

This is more commonly known simply as phlebitis and basically means an irritation within the veins of the legs that can result in blood clots which can then be transported to the heart or the brain, resulting in a stroke.

(5) ARTERIOSCLEROTIC VASCULAR DISEASE WITH EVIDENCE OF CIRCULATORY OBSTRUCTION.

This is fairly straightforward. If you have hardening of the arteries and your circulatory function is compromised because of an obstruction, you cannot safely fly.

(c) PERIPHERAL EDEMA.

This refers to swelling around the ankles, not secondary to injury. It is also sometimes noted in the fingers. This swelling, or edema, is of no concern by itself but usually indicates that there is something else going on, such as poor circulation or heart failure. The doctor will want to check further.

(d) SYNCOPE, THREATENED OR ACTUAL, DURING EXAMINATION.

Syncope is the same as fainting. Most people do not faint unless they are subjected to extremely stressful physical or emotional situations. For example, some pilots are sensitive to being stuck with needles, but the actual act of fainting could indicate some other underlying disorder. Therefore, this must be evaluated to rule out a disorder that would not be compatible with flying. This is an example of a condition on which the FAA, if provided with adequate documentation and evaluation, can come up with a favorable decision. However, the FAA cannot make this kind of a decision based only on a very simple statement from a doctor, such as: "This is only a fainting spell and of no consequence." The FAA must have valid medical data to make that conclusion.

(e) ANEURYSM OR ATERIOVENOUS FISTULA.

An aneurysm is a ballooning out of an artery, which then can "blow out" because of the weakness of the thin, stretched artery wall. The fistula is a connection between an artery and a vein and greatly decreases the efficiency of the circulatory system; blood will bypass an organ through that fistula instead of providing that organ with needed oxygen.

ITEM 38—ABDOMEN AND VISCERA (the internal organs of the abdomen such as the stomach, liver, pancreas, spleen, etc.)

(a) CHOLELITHIASIS (gall stones)

Although they may not be symptomatic, some doctors believe that the mere presence of gall stones can lead to a potentially severe attack that would be totally disabling. Such an attack might not occur, but because if could, the *presence* of gall stones is disqualifying. Once they are removed, you're OK.

(b) HEPATITIS, ACUTE; OR CHRONIC, WITH EVIDENCE OF IMPAIRMENT OF LIVER FUNCTION.

An active liver infection or an old infection that has left you with poor liver function is disqualifying. Anyone with hepatitis doesn't want to fly anyway.

(c) CIRRHOSIS.

This is *scarring* of the liver from any number of reasons, the more common cause being hepatitis and alcohol. Cirrhosis can occur in different degrees of severity and the individual is usually too sick to be flying. Less-severe cirrhosis would be certifiable providing it did not create any medical problems and was not progressive. Cirrhosis is a bad disease, and since it is usually associated with other problems, it is not easily certified.

(d) INGUINAL OR FEMORAL HERNIA IF OF A TYPE LIKELY TO BECOME INCARCERATED OR STRANGULATED.

A hernia is a weakness in the wall of the abdomen through which internal abdominal organs *can* protrude under pressure. Inguinal means in the groin. Femoral is basically the same area but a different type. The point is that the hernia could be big enough to potentially cause "strangulation" of the protruding organs, resulting in a medical emergency.

(e) HIATAL HERNIA IF SYMPTOMATIC.

Hiatus hernia is a hernia of the part of the stomach forced through the diaphragm of the abdomen where the esophagus passes through it. This is a relatively common finding, sometimes noted only by x-ray, but occasionally associated with disabling symptoms. However, if this is just an incidental finding and does not create any severe symptoms, there is no problem in certification.

(f) VENTRAL HERNIA.

This is an opening or weakness of the wall in the portion around the umbilicus or along the midline of the abdomen. The same reasoning prevails that there could be a potential strangulation of the internal contents of the abdomen.

(g) SPLENOMEGALY.

This means enlargement of the spleen and it, by itself, is of no consequence. There is the danger of injury during abdominal trauma because of its large size. But the problem here is the underlying *cause* of the enlarged spleen, such as a severe infection, cancer, etc. It is the cause of the splenomegaly that is of concern.

(h) INTRA-ABDOMINAL TUMORS OR MASSES.

Appendix II

Tumors and masses, until proven otherwise, are potentially dangerous.
- (i) SURGERY:
  - (1) GASTRIC RESECTION;
  - (2) SURGERY FOR MALIGNANCY;
  - (3) OTHER MAJOR SURGERY IF EVIDENCE OF INTERFERENCE WITH FUNCTION OR NUTRITION.
- (j) GASTRIC OR DUODENAL ULCER:
  - (1) ACTIVE: AN APPLICANT WITH EVIDENCE OR HISTORY OF AN ACTIVE ULCER WITHIN 3 MONTHS PRECEDING THE DATE OF EXAMINATION WILL BE REQUIRED TO PROVIDE EVIDENCE THAT THE ULCER IS HEALED BEFORE ANY CLASS OF MEDICAL CERTIFICATE IS ISSUED. EVIDENCE OF HEALING WILL BE ESTABLISHED BY A REPORT FROM THE ATTENDING PHYSICIAN TO INCLUDE STATEMENTS CONCERNING THE FOLLOWING:
    - (a) CONFIRMATION THAT THE APPLICANT HAS BEEN FREE OF SYMPTOMS.
    - (b) RADIOGRAPHIC EVIDENCE OF HEALING, UNLESS CONTRAINDICATED.
    - (c) TREATMENT, IN DETAIL, INCLUDING PRESENT MEDICATION.

    Ulcers have a tendency to recur unless totally resolved. An active ulcer can be very disabling and therefore is not compatible with flying. It must be proven that the ulcer is resolved. The use of medication, of course, is disqualifying, as stated before, and also implies that the ulcer *requires* medication to keep it under control.
  - (2) BLEEDING:

    A bleeding ulcer is a medical *emergency* and requires immediate attention. Bleeding ulcers have a great tendency to recur, and are a more severe medical problem than nonbleeding ulcers, which are more painful but less dangerous. Obviously, these ulcers require a more closely monitored follow-up program for the FAA.

ITEM 39 — ANUS AND RECTUM.
- (a) ACUTE OR CHRONIC INFECTION WHICH COULD RESULT IN INCAPACITY.
- (b) EVIDENCE OF RECTAL OR PROSTATIC MALIGNANCY.

    This part of the anatomy is important to *male* pilots because the prostate gland can become infected or inflamed. The presence of an infection, as with any serious infection, is disabling.

ITEM 40 — ENDOCRINE SYSTEM.

(a) **DIABETES MELLITUS** (Explained in the mandatory denials.)

(d) **DIABETES INSIPIDUS.**

This is a rare form of diabetes, usually the result of a more-serious endocrine system disorder. Anyone who has this disease is not fit to fly, nor would he really want to.

(c) **HYPERTHYROIDISM IF SYMPTOMATIC OR UNDER TREATMENT.**

*Hyper*thyroidism implies an overactive thyroid and the therapy for this is far more extensive than for the following, *hypo*thyroidism. It is also called Grave's Disease and used to be quite common in the Midwest. The complications of someone having hyperthyroidism can be very serious. Once again, however, anyone with severe hyperthyroidism, requiring therapy, usually is not well enough to fly anyway.

(d) **HYPOTHYROIDISM IF SYMPTOMATIC.** (Underactive thyroid)

Note that it doesn't say you cannot be under treatment. This means that the FAA will accept known *hypo*thyroidism if it is under medication — usually a supplemental thyroid hormone. Once you have been on this medication for a period of time and show no symptoms, you can be certified.

(e) **ADDISON'S DISEASE OR SYNDROME.**

(f) **CUSHING'S DISEASE OR SYNDROME.**

These are uncommon diseases of the endocrine glands that are as complex as diabetes, with a multitude of disabling results which are not compatible with flying.

(g) **HYPOGLYCEMIA: FUNCTIONAL OR DUE TO TUMOR OF PANCREAS.**

Hypoglycemia (low blood sugar) caused by a tumor, although rare, is easily diagnosed with additional tests. The symptoms are directly related to the tumor. However, "functional" hypoglycemia is very subjective. It is a "fad" illness influenced by the amount of publicity it receives in the papers and magazines. It is more closely related to a person's eating habits and his psychological makeup than to any disease process.

ITEM 41 — GENITOURINARY SYSTEM

(a) **CALCULUS:**
  (1) **RENAL, IF SMALL OR IF THERE IS ALTERATION OF RENAL FUNCTION.**
  (2) **URETERAL.**
  (3) **VESICAL IF LARGE AND SYMPTOMATIC.**

Calculus is the same as a small stone. Although usually not larger than a piece of sand, it can create extreme pain. If

Appendix II

the stone is found to be within the kidney (usually only determined by x-ray) and appears small enough that it might pass on through to the bladder, or if it is large enough to cause a change in the function of the kidney, then it is disqualifying. If it is in the ureter (a tube between the kidney and the bladder) or is vesicular (within the bladder itself) it can suddenly become very painful and can develop without warning. Anyone who has passed a kidney stone will attest that this is one of the most excruciating pains known to man. The chance of this occurring is related to the location and *presence* of the calculus or stone. A thorough evaluation is necessary.

(b) NEPHRECTOMY, IF ASSOCIATED WITH HYPERTENSION, UREMIA, INFECTION OF REMAINING KIDNEY, OR OTHER EVIDENCE OF REDUCED RENAL FUNCTION IN THE REMAINING KIDNEY.

Nephrectomy is the actual removal of a kidney. The regulation states that if the remaining kidney has any reduced function ("renal" indicating "kidney") then your over-all kidney function is severely compromised and not compatible with flying.

(c) NEPHRITIS, ACUTE OR CHRONIC.
(d) NEPHROSIS REGARDLESS OF ETIOLOGY.
(e) HYDRONEPHROSIS ASSOCIATED WITH IMPAIRMENT OF RENAL FUNCTION.
(f) PYONEPHROSIS.
(g) PYELITIS AND PYELONEPHRITIS.
(h) POLYCYSTIC DISEASE OF KIDNEYS.

All of these are diseases of the kidney and, although uncommon, can lead to decreased kidney function and therefore decrease your ability to metabolize properly. The degree of severity, as in any illness, has a great effect on whether it would interfere with your flying. Therefore, as mentioned several times earlier, you would be judged on the severity and the extent of the disease process. These disorders are definitely not safe to fly with if severe enough to cause you to be ill.

(i) OTHER ACTIVE RENAL DISEASE RESULTING IN INTERFERENCE WITH NORMAL FUNCTION.

This kidney has to function properly in order for you to function properly.

(j) TUMORS IF MALIGNANT OR INTERFERE WITH FUNCTION, OR LIKELY TO INTERFERE WITH FUNCTION.

As stated before, tumors shouldn't be there and can interfere if not resolved.

ITEM 42—UPPER AND LOWER EXTREMITIES

(a) AMPUTATION OF ANY EXTREMITY OR ANY PORTION THEREOF SUFFICIENT TO INTERFERE WITH THE PERFORMANCE OF AIRMAN DUTIES.

(b) ATROPHY (shrinking or weakening) OF MUSCLES OF ANY PART WHICH IS PROGRESSIVE OR IS SUFFICIENT TO INTERFERE WITH THE PERFORMANCE OR AIRMAN DUTIES.

(c) DEFORMITIES, EITHER CONGENITAL OR ACQUIRED: E.G., AS A RESULT OF MALUNION OF FRACTURE, ANKYLOSIS (stiffness) OF JOINTS, OR TRAUMA; IF SUFFICIENT TO INTERFERE WITH THE PERFORMANCE OF AIRMAN DUTIES.

(d) LIMITATION OF MOTION OF A MAJOR JOINT, IF SUFFICIENT TO INTERFERE WITH THE PERFORMANCE OF AIRMAN DUTIES.

(e) NEURALGIA (discomfort or strange sensation such as severe tingling or numbness), CHRONIC OR ACUTE, PARTICULARLY SCIATIC, IF IT RESULTS IN INTERFERENCE WITH FUNCTION OR IS LIKELY TO BECOME INCAPACITATING.

All of these are self-explanatory, especially where it states "interfere with the performance of airman duties." To be medically certified, you must be able to demonstrate your flying ability to an FAA flight examiner. This "demonstrated ability" results in a waiver for that defect, providing you pass.

(f) OSTEOMYELITIS, ACUTE OR CHRONIC, WITH OR WITHOUT DRAINING FISTULA.

Osteomyelitis is a severe inflammation of the bone. It can lead to chronic problems, is difficult to treat, is very painful, and is not compatible with flying. A fistula is a hole leading from the bone to the outside.

(g) TREMORS, IF OF SUFFICIENT DEGREE TO INTERFERE WITH THE PERFORMANCE OF AIRMAN DUTIES.

ITEM 43 — SPINE, OTHER MUSCULOSKELETAL

(a) ACTIVE DISEASE OF BONES AND JOINTS, INCLUDING ARTHRITIS.

Any disease of the bones and joints usually is disabling and painful enough that you wouldn't feel like flying anyway. However, arthritis can occur in various forms of severity. Most of us have experienced it in some degree at some time. Arthritis, in this instance, is meant to be either severe enough that it is disabling or of the chronic form, such as rheumatoid arthritis.

(b) CURVATURE, ANKYLOSIS, OR OTHER MARKED DEFORMITY OF THE SPINAL COLUMN SUFFICIENT TO IN-

TERFERE WITH THE PERFORMANCE OF AIRMAN DUTIES.
(c) HERNIATION OF INTERVERTEBRAL DISC.

This means a slipped disc. Notice that it does not say you cannot fly *after* it has been corrected. In other words, if you have a slipped disc or herniated disc, you probably have symptoms. This defect can also lead to progressive destruction of the nerve supply to the surrounding organs and limbs. Therefore, if it is not corrected, it can disqualify you. Once it is corrected, however, there is no problem being certified, provided you didn't wait too long for therapy.

(d) OTHER DISTURBANCES OF MUSCULOSKELETAL FUNCTION, CONGENITAL OR ACQUIRED, SUFFICIENT TO INTERFERE WITH THE PERFORMANCE OF AIRMAN DUTIES OR LIKELY TO PROGRESS TO THAT DEGREE.
  (1) MUSCULOSKELETAL EFFECTS OF CEREBRAL PALSY.
  (2) MYASTHENIA GRAVIS.
  (3) MUSCULAR DYSTROPHY OR OTHER MYOPATHIES.

  These are all self-explanatory. Myasthenia graves is a disease where the muscles are in a constantly relaxed condition and therefore do not function properly. Cerebral palsy and muscular dystrophy are well-known and obviously are not compatible with flying. Myopathy means any disease of the muscles that ultimately would disable a person.

ITEM 44—IDENTIFYING BODY MARKS, SCARS, AND TATTOOS. SCAR OR SCAR TISSUE WHICH INVOLVES THE FUNCTION OF STRUCTURES SUFFICIENT TO INTERFERE WITH SAFE PERFORMANCE OF AIRMAN DUTIES.

ITEM 45—SKIN, LYMPHATICS
(a) NEUROFIBROMATOSIS (VON RECKLINGHAUSEN'S DISEASE) IF ASSOCIATED WITH CONCOMITANT INVOLVEMENT OF CENTRAL NERVOUS SYSTEM.

This is a very uncommon skin disease, and if you had it, you wouldn't want to fly anyway.

(b) MALIGNANT MELANOMA OR, IF REMOVED, EVIDENCE OF METASTASIS.

Keep in mind here that if the melanoma (a skin tumor) has been removed and there is no sign of spread, you are certifiable.

(c) HODGKIN'S DISEASE, LYMPHOMA, LYMPHOSARCOMA.

Pilots have been certified after having these diseases, assuming, of course, that they have been resolved totally and there is little or no chance of continued spread or interference with normal body function.

(d) ADENOPATHY SECONDARY TO SYSTEMIC DISEASE OR METASTASIS.

Adenopathy means a swelling of the "glands," mainly the lymph nodes, and is an indication that there is either a systemic disease present that affects the whole body, or a metastasis (the spread of a malignancy) that is not controlled. It potentially can interfere with normal body function and therefore is not compatible with flying.

ITEM 46—NEUROLOGIC

(a) HISTORY OR FINDINGS SUGGESTING ANY OF THE FOLLOWING OCCURRENCES WILL REQUIRE FURTHER STUDY.
- (1) HEAD INJURY ASSOCIATED WITH LOSS OF CONSCIOUSNESS OF ONE HOUR OR MORE IN DURATION.
- (2) BRAIN SURGERY.

    These are self-explanatory, especially if the injury and surgery are severe enough to interfere with function as a pilot.

- (3) SUBARACHNOID HEMORRHAGE.

    In lay terms, this is the same as a stroke. It means that there has been bleeding within the brain. This is a medical emergency. The problem is in determining whether, after this has cleared, there will be a recurrence. In other words, unless there is a specific known cause for the bleeding and it has been corrected, a person who has had a subarachnoid hemorrhage has a far greater chance of a recurrence than someone who has not had an incident. Time often is the main factor in determining the probability of a recurrence. In some cases, the source of the bleeding is not found and therefore, without a cure, no one can really anticipate what the chances are for another occurrence.

- (4) CEREBRAL ANEURYSM.

    This is like a time bomb, an accident waiting for a time and place to happen. This usually has no symptoms and is found incidentally during the workup of another problem, such as severe headaches or an unexplained disturbance of consciousness. Once the aneurysm has been found or noted to be present, it must be cared for surgically before your consideration for flying status.

- (5) CEREBROVASCULAR DISEASE, INCLUDING CEREBROVASCULAR ACCIDENT.

    Any disease involving the blood vessels to the brain can be potentially severe enough to incapacitate a pilot. Cere-

Appendix II

brovascular accident is, again, the same as a stroke and the concern of the FAA is the probability of a recurrence.
(b) EPILEPSY. (Previously explained.)
(c) UNEXPLAINED DISTURBANCE OF CONSCIOUSNESS.

ITEM 47 — PSYCHIATRIC
(a) ESTABLISHED MEDICAL HISTORY OR CLINICAL DIAGNOSIS OF THE FOLLOWING WILL BE DISQUALIFYING.
   (1) CHARACTER OR BEHAVIOR DISORDER WHICH IS SUFFICIENTLY SEVERE TO HAVE REPEATEDLY MANIFESTED ITSELF BY OVERT ACTS.
   (2) CHRONIC ALCOHOLISM.
   (3) DRUG ADDICTION.
   (4) EPILEPSY.
   (5) PSYCHOTIC DISORDER.
(b) MENTAL DEFICIENCY.
   Mental deficiency is a very subjective finding and subject to much interpretation. This is not usually associated with professional pilots. It deals mainly with individuals who are classed as having severely low I.Q.'s.
(c) MENTAL DISORDERS REQUIRING CONTINUED OR INTERMITTENT MEDICATION.
   This category is actually a catch-all for any other mental disorder. The main point here is that a pilot with such a disorder cannot function without medication.
(d) PSYCHONEUROTIC DISORDERS WHICH RENDER OR COULD RENDER THE APPLICANT UNABLE SAFELY TO PERFORM THE DUTIES OF AN AIRMAN.
   (1) ANXIETY REACTION, ACUTE, CHRONIC, OR RECURRING.
   (2) OBSESSIVE-COMPULSIVE REACTIONS.
   (3) CONVERSION HYSTERIA.
   (4) DISSOCIATIVE REACTION.
   (5) DEPRESSIVE REACTION.
   (6) PHOBIC REACTION.
      These mental diseases are subject to interpretation as to severity and, as mentioned before, there is much skepticism as to how psychologists and psychiatrists can diagnose these problems and determine whether or not the "mental disorder" would interfere with flying. If it can be shown that a pilot who has one of these problems, such as depression or fears, can function properly and that these reactions would not interfere with his responsibility as a pilot, he could be certified. It is very important that the pilot have a physician evaluate these mental problems in light of future responsibil-

Pilot's Manual of Medical Certification

ities. It is possible that three different physicians could evaluate the same person and arrive at three different degrees of severity of illness and effect on flying. As was mentioned before, anyone who has one of these psychoneurotic disorders severe enough to interfere with his abilities to perform the duties of a pilot, even though it is not totally accepted or understood by that pilot and his peers, is definitely not certifiable. He is not safe in the air.

ITEM 48 — GENERAL SYSTEMIC

(a) BODY BUILD: ANY CONGENITAL OR ACQUIRED DEFECT WHICH WOULD ADVERSELY AFFECT FLYING SAFETY OR ENDANGER THE INDIVIDUAL'S WELLBEING IF PERMITTED TO FLY.

Note that obesity is not specifically mentioned. However, the fat pilot eventually will develop some other medical problem caused by being overweight that ultimately will interfere with his ability to fly and be certified.

(b) ANY ORGANIC OR FUNCTIONAL DISEASE OR STRUCTURAL DEFECT OR LIMITATION WHICH RENDERS OR COULD RENDER THE APPLICANT UNABLE SAFELY TO PERFORM THE DUTIES OF AN AIRMAN.

Once again, this is a catch-all to include diseases and problems not mentioned in the guide.

(c) MALIGNANCY:
   (1) LEUKEMIA AND OTHER BLOOD DYSCRASIAS.
   (2) MALIGNANT TUMOR OF ANY TYPE UNTIL COMPLETELY ERADICATED.

These were explained previously.

ITEM 49 — HEARING

(a) WHISPERED VOICE:

The whispered voice technique is a poor substitute for evaluation of your hearing ability. Although you can probably get by with very bad hearing through this technique, this is somewhat analogous to looking into the gas tank of a small aircraft to determine if it is one-third or one-half full and then deciding whether or not you've got enough gas to make the next leg. The only true way to monitor your hearing and to protect you from progressive problems such as exposure to noise is by using the audiometer. If you are having problems with your high frequency hearing, the only way this can be detected is through the audiometer. Your hearing could be in the process of being totally destroyed, a process which could be very easily stopped if you just knew that your high frequencies were failing. Without the audiometer reading, there is no way you can find out.

Appendix II

(b) AUDIOMETRIC:
  (1) CLASS I: HEARING LOSS GREATER THAN 40 DECIBELS IN EITHER EAR IN THE FREQUENCIES 500, AND 35 DECIBELS IN THE 1000 AND 2000 RANGE.

  A 35 decibel hearing loss is severe, yet it is acceptable. The frequencies of 500, 1000, and 2000 cycles per second include the normal voice range and the range used in your communication systems. The communication system is not a high-fidelity piece of equipment. Note that the FAA does not consider the frequencies above 2000 cycles per second. But it is in this high range (4000-8000 cycles per second) that you *first* will detect a decrease in your over-all hearing. This loss usually is a result of exposure to excessive noise, the most common cause of hearing loss. In most cases, someone with hearing loss in excess of 35 db has been able to adapt and can hear adequately. Therefore, waivers are very common for hearing losses in excess of 35 db, provided that the pilot still can perform. However, if his hearing loss is severe enough that he is unable to detect changes in the sound of his flying equipment that could be suggestive of a malfunction, or if he would miss communications or instructions from air traffic controllers or his cockpit colleagues, then this hearing loss obviously is not compatible with safe flying.

ITEM 50 — DISTANT VISION
(a) CLASSES I AND II: UNCORRECTED ACUITY POORER THAN 20/100 IN EITHER EYE. UNCORRECTED ACUITY POORER THAN 20/20 IN EITHER EYE NOT CORRECTABLE TO AT LEAST 20/20.

  This was described in the section on the Federal Air Regulations.

ITEM 51 — NEAR VISION
(a) CLASSES I AND II: FAILURE TO DEMONSTRATE AN ACCOMMODATION OF AT LEAST 20/40 WITH EACH EYE SEPARATELY WITH OR WITHOUT CORRECTION.

  This also was described previously.

ITEM 52 — INTRAOCULAR TENSION
(a) GLAUCOMA
(b) APPARENT INCREASED TENSION

ITEM 53 — COLOR VISION

ITEM 54 — FIELD OF VISION

  Refer to Chapter 7 for items 52-54.

ITEM 55 — HETEROPHORIA
(a) DIPLOPIA: ALL CLASSES

  Diplopia means double vision. It obviously is incompatible with safe flying.

(b) SUPPRESSION SUFFICIENT TO PREVENT DETERMINATION OF HETEROPHORIA.

Suppression means that you have a "lazy eye" (or a weak eye) causing so much deviation in your ability to fuse your vision that the lazy eye no longer can see well. Thus, the ability to see with both eyes equally is suppressed.

(c) HETEROPHORIA
CLASSES I AND II:
  (1) HYPERPHORIA GREATER THAN 1-PRISM DIOPTER.
  (2) ESOPHORIA GREATER THAN 6-PRISM DIOPTERS.
  (3) EXOPHORIA GREATER THAN 6-PRISM DIOPTERS.

Normal use of the muscles that move the eyes enables you to look at an object with both eyes and "see" it, as interpreted by the brain, as a singular image. Heterophoria is the tendency of the eyes to move away from the correct focused position, especially when tired or fatigued, resulting in images that are not fused. One eye will have a tendency to "drift" and a double image occurs. Hyperphoria, esophoria, and exophoria indicate the direction that the eye is drifting. Even though you may not meet the standards of the FAA, your ability to pass a flight test and a further evaluation by a doctor could lead to a waiver.

ITEM 56—BLOOD PRESSURE
(a) ELEVATED BLOOD PRESSURE
  (1) CLASS I:

This was noted earlier in our discussion of the actual regulations. The specific subject of blood pressure was discussed in Chapter 7.

  (2) CLASSES II AND III: BLOOD PRESSURE ABOVE 170 mm. OF MERCURY SYSTOLIC OR 100 mm. OF MERCURY DIASTOLIC.
  (3) ALL CLASSES: CONTINUING MEDICATION FOR TREATMENT OF HIGH BLOOD PRESSURE, REGARDLESS OF LEVEL OF PRESSURE.

This simply means that if you have blood pressure that requires medication, then it can be assumed that all other techniques have been tried and were unsuccessful. You are not qualified to fly until this situation has been completely evaluated.

ITEM 57—PULSE
(a) PULSE RATE OF MORE THAN 100 BEATS PER MINUTE AT REST.
(b) PULSE RATE OF MORE THAN 120 BEATS PER MINUTE IMMEDIATELY AFTER EXERCISE.

Appendix II

(c) FAILURE OF PULSE RATE TO RETURN AFTER 2 MINUTES TO WITHIN 20 BEATS OF THE LEVEL OF THE RESTING PULSE.

These values are used as a guide and are not absolute. An airman who comes to an aviation medical examiner often is anxious or even scared and naturally his pulse will go up. The interpretation of the examining physician is very important at this state of his examination. No pilot should be grounded simply because of an "abnormal" pulse rate.

(d) IRREGULARITIES OTHER THAN OCCASIONAL SKIPPED BEAT OR SINUS ARRYTHMIA.

An irregular pulse sometimes is an indication of an abnormal heart function. It requires further elaboration and more information than normally gained by an FAA exam. Sinus arrhythmia is a type of heart rhythm irregularity. These irregularities can be benign or significant and therefore require further tests.

(e) DEVELOPMENT OF AN EPISODE OF TACHYCARDIA IN THE COURSE OF EXAMINATION.

Tachycardia is a rapid *resting* pulse rate. Rapid usually means in excess of 120 beats per minute. This is not the usual finding, even under the stress of the examination. It usually is an indication of some abnormal heart function and requires further evaluation, especially if the pulse changes abruptly to a high rate.

(f) PULSE RATE LOWER THAN 50 BEATS PER MINUTE.

Obviously, this does not pertain to the jogger or long-distance runner. However, pulse that slow in someone who is not a jogger is significant and, again, may indicate some other heart problem. It then requires further evaluation.

ITEM 58 — URINALYSIS

(a) PROTEINURIA, UNTIL ABSENCE OF DISQUALIFYING SYSTEMIC OR GENITOURINARY CONDITIONS HAS BEEN DEMONSTRATED.

Proteinuria means protein in the urine which is not supposed to be there. It may indicate kidney disease. However, this occurrence often is associated with exercise or an acceptable variation of metabolism. Nevertheless, it requires further evaluation and should be checked before submitting the application to the FAA.

(b) GLYCOSURIA.

This means sugar in the urine and, until proven otherwise, is an indication of the possibility of diabetes. Diabetes is explained in Chapter 7.

ITEM 59 — ELECTROCARDIOGRAM

(a) ARRHYTHMIAS, EXCEPT SINUS ARRHYTHMIA AND OCCASIONAL VENTRICULAR EXTRASYSTOLE.

Arrhythmia means irregular rhythm and the same as mentioned in Item 57, paragraph (d). This relates to the findings on the electrocardiographic tracing, not determined by *feeling* your pulse.
(b) CONDUCTION DEFECTS SUCH AS: (Conduction defects are interruptions in the normal electrical impulse pattern that produces a heartbeat.)
    (1) COMPLETE HEART BLOCK.
        This can be a severe heart problem, especially when associated with stress and low oxygen availability when flying at altitude. The conduction defects, unfortunately, are not often picked up until an electrocardiogram is done and, therefore, catch the applicant by surprise since he usually is without symptoms. Simply being free of symptoms does not guarantee good health.
    (2) LEFT BUNDLE BRANCH BLOCK.
        Left bundle branch block is another abnormality shown in the EKG tracing that gives no symptoms to the applicant. The left bundle branch block has, in some cases, a higher incidence of potential heart problems and therefore requires further evaluation.
    (3) RIGHT BUNDLE BRANCH BLOCK ASSOCIATED WITH CONGENITAL OR ORGANIC HEART DISEASE.
        The right bundle branch block is less-severe in nature than the left bundle, unless it is associated with some other heart problem.
    (4) WOLFF-PARKINSON-WHITE SYNDROME.
        This is a finding on an EKG and is also asymptomatic to the applicant. In some cases it is indicative of other heart problems. All these "conduction" defects are difficult to understand for the applicant who has no symptoms, is in good shape and who may even be an active jogger. As will be described later, it is not the mere presence of the finding that is significant but what it represents in the heart and what it could potentially become in the environment of flying.
(c) UNEQUIVOCAL ELECTROCARDIOGRAPHIC EVIDENCE OF
    (1) MYOCARDIAL INFARCTION, RECENT OR OLD. (A heart attack.)
    (2) CORONARY ARTERY DISEASE.
    (3) VENTRICULAR STRAIN.
    (4) VENTRICULAR HYPERTROPHY.
        (1) and (2) are already explained. Ventricular strain and ventricular hypertrophy mean somewhat the same

thing, in that the heart has to work harder than it normally should because the heart is out of shape or diseased. This is also subject to interpretation by the examiner and the FAA and requires further data to evaluate it.

EXPLANATION OF REMAINING PORTION OF FAA FORM 8500

ITEMS 60 — OTHER TESTS

THE NEED FOR ADDITIONAL MEDICAL EXAMINATIONS WILL BE DETERMINED FROM THE EXAMINER'S FINDINGS. EXAMINERS ARE AUTHORIZED TO REQUEST SUPPLEMENTARY EXAMINATIONS CONSISTING OF LABORATORY TESTS OR EXAMINATION BY APPROPRIATE MEDICAL SPECIALISTS. THE APPLICANT WILL BE ADVISED CONCERNING THE TYPES OF ADDITIONAL EXAMINATIONS REQUIRED AND THE TYPE OF MEDICAL SPECIALIST TO BE CONSULTED FOR FURTHER EXAMINATION. RESONSIBILITY FOR ASSURING THE FORWARDING OF REPORTS OF THESE EXAMINATIONS AND FOR PAYMENT OF CHARGES WILL REST WITH THE APPLICANT. ALL REPORTS WILL BE FORWARDED TO THE AEROMEDICAL CERTIFICATION BRANCH, OKLAHOMA CITY, OKLAHOMA.

This is self-explanatory, but note that the applicant is entitled to know the reason for the additional tests. Also note that the responsibility for making sure the additional reports are submitted is with the *applicant* and not the medical examiner.

Index

A

Abdomen, 153
Additives, 94
Aerobic exercises, 99
Aeromedical advisor, 53
Aeromedical certification branch, 33, 139, 167
Aeromedical Coordinator, 51
Aeromedical physician, 14, 17, 51
Aerospace medicine, 83
Age 60 Retirement Rule, 19
Airline Pilots Association, 51
Albumin, 36
Alcohol, 124, 126
Alcoholism, 21
Allergies, 149
ALPA, 21
AME, 12, 14, 15, 25, 26, 28, 30 35 36 37, 40, 43, 45, 46, 51, 83, 84, 140
Amino acids, 87
Amputation, 158
Anemia, 151
Anemias, 93
Aneurysm, 153, 160
Angiogram, 23
Angina pectoris, 23, 135, 150
Antihistamines, 70, 126
Anus & rectum, 155
Anxiety, 161
Applicant, 37, 167
Application, 26, 52
Arrhythmia, 151, 165, 166
Arthritis, 158
Asthma, 149
Atherosclerosis, 93
Audiogram, 36, 69
Audiometer, 133, 162
Aviation doctors, 82
Aviation medical examiner, 11, 19
Aviation medicine, 14

B

Bifocals, 66
Bleeding, 155
Bleeding ulcer, 155

Blindness, 13
Blood Pressure, 16, 17, 36, 41, 52, 56, 57, 64, 71, 81, 118, 119, 127, 136, 164
Blood vessels, 145
Board of Doctors, 54
Board of Specialists, 53
Bypass surgery, 65
Bulk, 127

C

Caffeine, 123
Calories, 98, 99, 100, 101, 102, 111, 112, 115, 117
  empty, 113
Carbohydrates, 98, 99, 111
Cardiac stress testing, 65
Cardiovascular evaluation, 24, 60, 75, 136
CAT scan, 23
Cataracts, 132, 145
Cellulose, 100
Certifiable, 78
Certificate, 34, 40
Certification, 84
Certify, 27, 28, 33, 44
Character or behavior disorder, 20
Chest X-ray, 71
Cholesterol, 63, 64, 94, 103
  elevated, 23
Cigarettes, 77
Cigarette smoking, 64
Cirrhosis, 154
Coffee, 125, 126, 127
Colds & flu, 128
"Color blindness", 67
"Color Threshold Test", 67
Color vision deficiency, 41, 67
Color vision, 132
Common medical factors, 56
Company aviation doctors, 82, 83
Company benefits, 14
Complete physicals, 21
Concussion, 22
Constipation, 127

Index

Consultants, 52
Contact lenses, 41, 66
Convulsion, 22
Convulsive disorder, 134
Coronary angiogram, 73
Coronary arteries, 23, 73, 122
Coronary artery disease, 23, 56, 63, 64, 166
Coronary heart disease, 23, 150
Correspond, 33

D

Decongestants, 70
Denials, 46, 63, 65, 146
Dehydrated, 57, 104
Dehydration, 124, 125, 126, 127
Depression, 161
Depth perception, 67
Diabetes, 24, 36, 56, 61, 93, 165
Diabetes Mellitus, 137, 156
Diarrhea, 127
Diet, 24, 62
   diabetic, 62
   fad, 15, 114, 115
   hocus-pocus, 111
   "miracle", 94
Dietary, 57
Disqualify, 30
Disqualifying conditions, 37
Disqualifying disorders, 28
Distant vision, 163
Distant visual activity, 131
Disturbance of consciousness, 22, 134
Diuretic, 124, 125
Dizziness, 143
Drug, 18, 21, 22
Drug addiction, 21

E

Ear, 133, 143
Ear block, 69, 127
Eardrum, 133, 144
Ear wax, 70, 144
EKG, 23, 35, 71, 72, 73, 76
Electrocardiogram, 165, 166
Electrocardiographic examination, 135
Emphysema, 122, 147
Enlarged heart, 150
Epilepsy, 22, 134
Eustachian Tube, 70, 144
Eyes, 144
Excessive noise, 69
Exercise, 115
Exercise apparatus, 121
Exercise and cardiac stress, 24
"Executive" physical, 37
Exemption, 21

Exemption process, 44
Exemption to FARS, 53
Evaluation components, 86

F

FAA's Cardiac stress testing, 71
FAA's cardiovascular evaluation, 71
FAA criteria, 14
FAA doctors, 12, 34, 35, 52
FAA exam, 6
FAA examiner, 77
FAA physical, 30
FAA Form 8500-8, 26, 30, 35, 36, 37, 40, 46, 51, 140
FAA health monitoring program, 8
FAA involvement, 10
Fainting, 153
Family doctor, 53, 77, 78, 83
FAR 91.11, 21
   91.11 (a) (3), 18, 125
   61.53, 18, 24, 30, 43, 44, 26, 89, 140
FAR 67, 19 Special issue, 21
   Part 67.19c, 55
   Part 67, 19, 25, 89
   Part 121, 19
   Part 61.53, 19
"Fasting" blood sugar, 62
Fast food, 93
Fatigability, 123
Fatigue, 214, 125, 126, 127
Fatiguing noise, 69, 126
Fats, 96, 98, 100, 102, 111
Fatty acids, 103
Federal Air Surgeon, 12, 20, 25, 27, 34, 44, 52, 53, 135, 137, 138, 139
Fiber, 101
First aid on trip, 127
Flight surgeons, 11, 14, 15, 45, 141
Flight tests, 67
Food fadists, 94

G

Gall stones, 153
Genitourinary system, 156
Glasses, 41, 65
Glaucoma, 12, 13, 36, 66, 145, 163
Glucose, 100
Glucose tolerance, 62
"Grounded" (not flying), 18, 24, 25, 30, 34, 33, 44, 64, 77, 80, 83, 84, 89, 90, 124, 129
Guide for Aviation Medical Examiners, 17, 25

H

Hayfever, 141

169

Health maintenance program, 9, 14, 55, 76, 77, 84, 87, 90, 114
Healthy, 24, 25
Hearing, 41, 68, 162
   ability, 36
   acuity, 133
   loss, 69, 163
   test, 36
Heart, 150
   attack, 19, 23, 43, 63, 104, 166
   block, 166
   disease, 93, 94
   failure, 64, 151
   muscle, 63, 117, 124
Hemorrhoids, 128
Hepatitis, 154
Hernia, 154
High blood pressure, 17, 23, 56, 73, 74
   common causes, 59
   control of, 60
Hodgkins Disease, 159
Hypertension, 17, 23, 57, 58, 59, 60, 65, 77, 93
Hyperthyroidism, 156
Hypoglycemia, 156
Hypoxia, 123
Hypoxic, 57

I

Inactivity, 127, 128
Incapacitate, 9
Insulin, 24, 137

J

Jog, 117
Jogging, 119

K

Kidney, 157
   stone, 157

L

Laboratory tests, 167
Lazy eye, 164
Left bundle branch block, 166
Leukemia, 152
Lungs and chest, 147
Limitations, 19
   functional, 40, 41, 55, 138, 139
   operational, 18, 40, 41
Letter of denial, 46, 52
Loss of license, 14

M

Malignancy, 162
Malignant tumor, 142
Mandatory (denial), 19, 20, 43, 53, 140

Masters Two-Step Stress Test, 72
"Mature onset" diabetes, 24
Medical certification, 15, 141
   first class, 18, 19, 23, 25, 30, 36, 55, 66
   second class, 19, 55, 67
   third class, 19, 38, 67
Medical criteria, 15
   deficiency, 18, 24
   departments, 51
   disorders, 19
   evaluations, 89, 138
   standards, 44
Medically screened, 5
Medication, 22, 24, 60, 61, 62, 77, 126, 128, 155, 156
   high blood pressure, 59
   over-the-counter, 125
Medicine, 84, 125
Megavitamins, 94
Mental disease, 20
Mental disorders, 133
Minerals, 96, 107, 108
Monitor, 10
   periodically, 5
Mouth and throat, 143
Murmur, 151
Mycocardial infarction, 22, 135

N

Narcotics, 22
Nasal sprays, 70
Near vision, 66, 131, 163
Neurologic, 160
Neurologic disorders, 134
Nephritis, 157
Night vision, 123
Nine mandatory disorders, 44
Nose, 141
NTSB (National Transportation Safety Board), 19, 54
Nutrients, 96, 101, 111
Nutritional cults, 94

O

Obese, 92
Obesity, 93, 162
Oklahoma City, 52, 83
   doctors, 12, 34
Operational experience, 138
   limitations, 4
Oral hypoglycemia, 24
Oral insulin, 24
"Ortho K", 68
Overweight, 100
Oxygen, 64

Index

P

Paranoid, 21
Pericarditis, 150
Personality disorders, 20, 134
Physicals, 26, 28
Physical condition, 24
Physical conditioning programs, 15
Physical fitness, 119
Physical examination, 36
Phlebitis, 153
Pilot in Command, 18
Pleurisy, 148
Practical test, 138
Preventive maintenance, 16
Pre-employment/company physical exams, 73
Prostate gland, 155
Protein, 96, 97, 100, 111
    sources, 97, 98
Psychiatric therapy, 20, 21
Psychiatrist, 127
Psychiatry, 21
Psychology, 21
Psychologist, 217
Psychotic disorder, 21
Pulse, 36, 90, 118, 120, 127, 164, 165
    resting, 117
    irregular, 165

R

Recommended Daily Allowances (RDA), 109
Rectal itching, 128
Reconsiderations, 19
Refractions, 66
Regional Flight Surgeon, 34, 43, 83, 139
Relaxation therapy, 126
REM sleep, 125
Renal glycosuria, 62
Retirement, 128
Right bundle branch block, 166
Risk, 28, 123, 142
Risk factors, 64, 71, 85, 86
Roughage, 101

S

"Schizophrenia", 21
Scuba diver, 71, 143
Self-grounded, 45
"Sick", 15, 27
Side Effects, 24, 126
Sinus block, 70, 142
Sinuses, 142
Slipped disk, 159
Smoking, 122
Sore legs, 128
"Space Myopia", 68
Special issue, 21
Special Medical Flight Test, 138
"Sphygmomanometer", 57
Spine, 158
Split personality, 21
ST segment, 72
Standards, 25
Stress, 57
Stress management, 127
Stress tests, 72
Stimulant, 123, 124
Stimulative, 124
Stroke, 43, 93, 104, 160, 161
Sugar, 36, 61, 94, 100
Supplementary evaluations, 46
Surgery, 155

T

Tachycardia, 165
Tests, 36, 167
Thalium scan, 23, 73
Time zone, 126
Tonometer, 13
Tonometry, 36, 66
Triglycerides, 64, 103
True health status, 86
Tumor, 142

U

Ulcer, 155
Union, 53
Urine, 36
Urinalysis, 61, 165
USAF flight surgeon, 18

V

Valsalva, 70, 142, 143, 144
Vascular system, 157
Vertigo, 143
Vision, 13, 36, 43, 65
Vision tests, 65
"Visual cues", 67
Vitamins, 96
    fat soluable, 102, 106
    water soluable, 105
    and minerals, 105

W

Waiver, 19, 41, 43, 149, 163
Water, 96, 124
Water Hydration, 104
Weight, 64
Weight control, 127
Weight loss, 77
Withdrawal, 125
Wolff-Parkinson-White Syndrome, 166
Working environment, 57

Richard O. Reinhart is Board Certified in family practice and specializes full time in aviation medicine and aeromedical certification in the Minneapolis area. He currently is a USAF Flight Surgeon with the Minnesota Air National Guard, a senior FAA AME, a rated scuba diver, and an instrument rated commercial pilot with a wide variety of experience in civilian and military aircraft. Dr. Reinhart is active in a variety of aeromedical and aviation organizations such as NBAA, AOPA, The Aerospace Medical Association, The Flying Physicians Assoc. The Minnesota Business Aircraft Assoc, etc. He is the aeromedical advisor for a major airline as well as several corporate flight departments and is a frequent speaker at various seminars sponsored by such organizations as Embry-Riddle Aeronautical University and the Departments of Transportation of Wisconsin and Minnesota. Dr. Reinhart also publishes an aeromedical newsletter for the aircrews he serves.

Also Published by Specialty Press

Reflections of Blue:
A Pictorial History of the U.S. Navy Blue Angles
Carol Knotts

Diamond in the Sky:
A Pictorial History of the USAF Thunderbirds
Carol Knotts and Pete Moore

The X Planes:
Experimental Aircraft from X-1 through X-29
Jay Miller

Harrier
Bill Gunston

F-15 Eagle
Jeff Ethell

Pilot Maker:
The Incredible T6
Walt Ohlrich and Jeff Ethell

Fighters of the Fifties
Bill Gunston

Delta Wings
Convair's High Speed Aircraft of the 1950's and 1960's
Charles Mendenhall

Deadly Duo:
The B25 and B26 in WWII
Charles Mendenhall

The Gee Bee Racers:
A Legacy of Speed
Charles Mendenhall

The Air Racer
Charles Mendenhall

Birkie Fever
A Ten Year History of the American Birkebeiner
Tom Kelly

Secrets of Buying and Selling Collector Cars
John Olson